U0217324

本项目获得北京市东城区优秀人才培养资助

Tuina Manipulation Atlas
of the Famous Senior TCM Doctor Cui Shusheng

名老中医崔述生推拿手法图谱

Study Group Led By Famous Senior TCM Doctor Cui Shusheng

崔述生名老中医工作室　编写

化学工业出版社

·北京·

图书在版编目（CIP）数据

名老中医崔述生推拿手法图谱=Tuina Manipulation Atlas of the Famous Senior TCM Doctor Cui Shusheng: 英文/ 崔述生名老中医工作室编写. —北京：化学工业出版社，2018.1

ISBN 978-7-122-31305-8

Ⅰ.①名… Ⅱ.①崔… Ⅲ.①推拿-图谱 Ⅳ.①R244.1-64

中国版本图书馆CIP数据核字（2017）第319521号

责任编辑：邱飞婵 吴 刚
责任校对：王素芹   装帧设计：关 飞

出版发行：化学工业出版社（北京市东城区青年湖南街13号 邮政编码100011）
印　　装：北京东方宝隆印刷有限公司
710mm×1000mm 1/16 印张12¾ 字数261千字 2018年4月北京第1版第1次印刷

购书咨询：010-64518888（传真：010-64519686） 售后服务：010-64518899
网　　址：http://www.cip.com.cn
凡购买本书，如有缺损质量问题，本社销售中心负责调换。

Work group of this book

Writers   Wang Yongqian   Sun Bo

Chief Translator   Geng Junlong

Collating workers   Li Dianbo   Meng Zhouling   Cui Xuan

Zhuang Minghui   Li Luguang   Wang Xinwei

Song Xiaojuan   Liu Dapeng

Counselor   Cui Shusheng

Models   Li Dianbo   Meng Zhouling   Song Xiaojuan

Photography   Wang Xing

【 FOREWORD 】

Chinese Tuina therapy is a science pertaining to the study of injuries to the skin, flesh, muscles, bones, qi, blood, zang-fu organs and meridians, at the same time it is a preventive method which can strengthen immunity and treat illnesses. Tuina is an essential aspect of traditional Chinese medicine with a long history of treating people of all ethnic groups and having significant results with pain. It has since become an independent subject with integrated theoretical systems. "Hands move along with thought and skills show up with the hands." Tuina, which is loosely translated into massage therapy in English, is a TCM clinical technology requiring first and foremost doctors' experiences and skills which are inherited from the masters through rigorous commitment. That is "the master may teach, but the progress is up to the hard work of the individual."

Mr. Cui Shusheng has been a disciple of three famous experts from Beijing: Liu Shoushan, Lu Yinghua and Ma Zaishan. For ten years, Dr.Cui Shusheng Learned from these masters. He has strictly followed the old maxim and has learned from all factions. He has practiced medicine for decades. At present he is over 60 years old, but his clinic is still crowded with patients. His therapeutic regimen is a combination of manipulations and medicine, wise and skilful, always having a masterful effect. Although he has profound skills, he prefers teaching, learning and practicing by himself. Because of he never hide his skills from others, his students are numerous and learn through clinical experiences. He proposes that in order to learn Tuina or massage therapy, one should improve both medical techniques and self-cultivation. He has compiled the "Tuina manipulations Atlas of the famous senior TCM doctor Cui Shusheng" with inherited skills and self-taught unique techniques which has withstood the difficulties of time. The Atlas is comprised with introductory skills, directing qi, application of strength, making difficult tasks simple and bringing forth the new through the old so as to help young students improve themselves and exchange experiences with their counterparts.

Being entrusted to make the foreword I am glad to finish it. "April showers bring May flowers". I hope that more scholars and counterparts can be benefit from this concise atlas written by Mr. Cui and more excellent works appear as well.

Written by Tu Zhitao

【 PREFACE 】

Tuina therapy, as an important part of traditional Chinese medicine and has a long history. It plays an irreplaceable role in the prevention and treatment of many diseases and is diversified by various factions, and different characteristic. This book is a collection of Professor Cui Shusheng's manual techniques as well as notations of his experience through clinical practice. The book includes effective manipulations in clinical practice as much as possible for amateurs practitioners to apply efficiently.

This book is divided into three parts:

Basic Tuina Manipulations: This chapter introduces the commonly used basic tuina manipulations, including definition, mechanism of action, operating positions, methods and attention points. Those tuina manipulations are widely used and applicable for most indications requiring tuina therapy.

Tuina Manipulations Applied on Different Part of the Body: This chapter includes 11 sections which introduce the tuina manipulations used on 10 parts of the body and the technique of pediatrics. Each section includes the basic tuina manipulations, special tuina techniques and clinical application. The basic tuina manipulations are common manipulations used in treatment of most illnesses occurring in relevant part of the body in clinic. The manipulations explained in the first chapter are not repeated here. Special tuina techniques are those used for some illnesses occurring in relevant part of the body. Clinical application provides some cases treated by Professor Cui Shusheng, and his manual techniques on specified diseases are summarized. This part includes the manipulations mentioned above, thus no atlas is provided.

Exercises for Manipulation Practice: This chapter mainly introduces Eighteen Exercises for practice, Baduanjin Exercise on the bed, and Relaxing Exercise for the cultivation of the tuina practitioner.

The diseases mentioned in the book involve traumatology diseases, orthopedic diseases, medical diseases, gynecological diseases, pediatric diseases, etc., thus it can be used clinically by medical working staff, used for both teaching and scientific research, and it can be consulted by amateurs as well. If there are any improper descriptions, please point them out so that they can be corrected.

The writing work of this book is done by the Study Group Led By Nationally-Acclaimed TCM Doctor Cui Shusheng. We would like to thank Ilyas Ambeyah Hamid and Jonathan M. Fields Ap from American for their arduous labor in the revision of this book.

The authors
August 2017 in Beijing,China

【 CONTENTS 】

Chapter 1　Basic Tuina Manipulations

Chapter 2　Tuina Manipulations Applied on Different Part of the Body

Chapter 3   Exercises for Manipulation Practice

Chapter 1

Basic Tuina Manipulations

1.1 Catapult-plucking manipulation

Catapulting refers to a manipulation performed by holding the affected muscle or tendon with the thumb and other fingers and immediately releasing it to make it catapult back. (Fig.1-1)

Plucking refers to the finger tips being pressed into the affected area deeply and plucking back and forth. The direction of the movement should be perpendicular to the direction of the tendon and muscle.

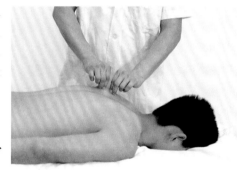

Fig.1-1   Catapulting Manipulation

The two manipulations can be used separately, together, and combined with kneading manipulation. The catapult-plucking manipulation refers primarily to the plucking technique. This manipulation works on muscle and tendon to relieve spasm. And it can also treat the numbness or pain of the limbs by working on the nerve trunks. During the manipulation, the force varies from slight to heavy, and the movement should be gentle and elastic. Repeat this operation several times as necessary.

Treatment requirements

Find the areas that need treatment and apply the right amount of force into the corresponding level, then pluck the tissues. The direction of the movement should be perpendicular to the direction of the tendon and muscle. The focus position must be driven by upper limb with the fixed metacarpophalangeal joints and interphalangeal joints to help the manipulator avoid injuring their joints. It also can prevent scratches on

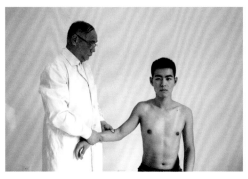

Fig.1-2　Plucking manipulation with the thumb

the patient's skin. The manipulators should use physics and leverage to gain strength by changing their positions to adapt to the regions being treated.

(1) *Plucking manipulation with the thumb*
Press the treatment area deeply with the thumb, lower the shoulder, drop the elbow, drive the thumb with upper limb, pluck back and forth perpendicular to the direction of the tendon and muscle. (Fig.1-2)

(2) *Plucking manipulation with overlapping thumbs*
The manipulator puts one thumb on the treatment area and overlaps the other thumb on it. Drive the thumbs with upper limbs, and pluck back and forth perpendicular to the direction of the tendon, muscle and stripe. (Fig.1-3)

(3) *Plucking manipulation with the elbow*
Lower shoulders and drop elbow with the wrist joint flexed naturally to about 90°. Press the treatment area deeply with olecranon, and pluck back and forth. Using the rotational motion of the shoulder, pluck left and right perpendicular to the direction of the tendon and muscle. The elbow plucking manipulation can be used together with pointing, kneading, and pressing. It should be performed softly and deeply to penetrate. (Fig.1-4)

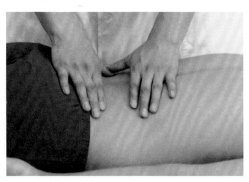

Fig.1-3　Plucking manipulation with overlapping thumbs

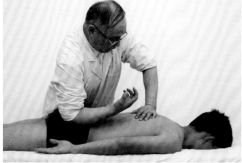

Fig.1-4　Plucking manipulation with the elbow

(4) *Plucking manipulation with the four fingers*
Press the treatment area deeply with the tip or whole surface of your four fingers and support with the thumb naturally. Lower the shoulder, drop the elbow, and drive the four fingers with upper limb. Pluck back and forth perpendicular to the direction of the tendon and muscle. This manipulation can be alternately used with the thumb plucking method

to avoid getting tired.(Fig.1-5)

The main applicable regions

Plucking manipulation with the thumb is mainly applied on the neck, shoulders and limbs. Plucking manipulation with overlapping thumbs is mainly applied on the back and waist. Plucking manipulation with the elbow is applied on the lower back and buttocks of those whose muscles are well developed. Plucking manipulation with four fingers is mainly applied on the neck and shoulders.

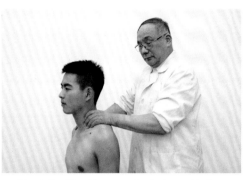

Fig.1-5   Plucking manipulation with four fingers

Cautions

The manipulator should pluck back and forth perpendicular to the direction of the tendon, muscle and stripe. The force used should be increased gradually and softly. To avoid further tissue damage, long time plucking of the affected region is prohibited. The practitioner can use it together with vibrating manipulation for the practician so that the force is deep and penetrative enough.

1.2   Rolling manipulation

Place the dorsal aspect of the hand or elbow over the treatment area and roll the forearm and dorsum of hand back and forth continuously. This is called rolling manipulation. It can promote blood circulation, relax the tendons, unblock the collaterals, relieve spasm, alleviate pain and relax tight, stiff and fatigued muscles.

Treatment requirements

When performing the rolling manipulation, fix on the affected area with the back of hand or forearm. The upper limb should remain relaxed. The frequency should be fixed and the speed should not too quick. The stimulation should be performed with light and heavy force alternately.

(1) *Elevated rolling manipulation*

Press the affected area with the dorsal aspect of proximal interphalangeal joints of the index, middle and ring fingers. Replace the complex rotation of the forearm with simple movement of extension and flexion of the wrist joint. The force and stimulation is stronger, so it is often applied to the areas with thick muscles on a person with strong physique. (Fig.1-6)

(2) *Side rolling manipulation*

With naturally-bent fingers and a relaxed upper limb, press with the dorsal aspect of the 5th metacarpophalangeal joint over the treatment area. Roll the hypothenar and dorsum of the hand back and forth continuously. The rolling movement is achieved by the flexion and extension of the wrist joint, coupled with a rotation of the forearm by using the elbow joint as a pivot. The force is slight and the stimulation is soft, so it is often applied to joints and on people with a small physique. (Fig.1-7; Fig.1-8)

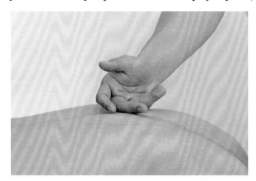

Fig.1-6　Elevated rolling manipulation　　　Fig.1-7　Side rolling manipulation Ⅰ

(3) *Forearm rolling manipulation*

With naturally-bent fingers in a claw shape and a relaxed shoulder, press the affected area with the ulnar side of forearm close to the elbow. Drop the elbow with the wrist joint flexed naturally to 90° and roll back and forth continuously. The forearm rotates outwards while swaying the arm externally, and inwards while swaying the arm backward. (Fig.1-9 to Fig.1-13)

The main applicable regions

This manipulation is often applied to the areas with thick muscles like shoulders, back, lower back and limbs.

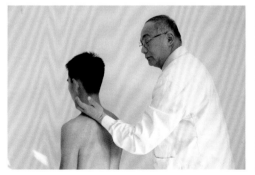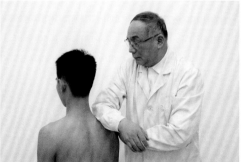

Fig.1-8　Side rolling manipulation Ⅱ　　　Fig.1-9　Forearm rolling manipulation Ⅰ

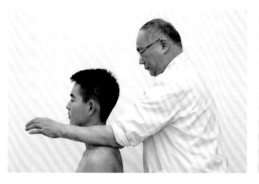

Fig.1-10　Forearm rolling manipulation Ⅱ

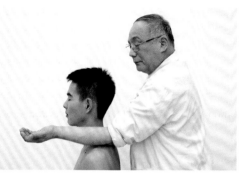

Fig.1-11　Forearm rolling manipulation Ⅲ

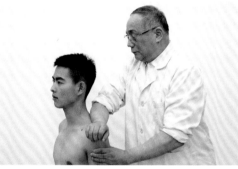

Fig.1-12　Forearm rolling manipulation Ⅳ

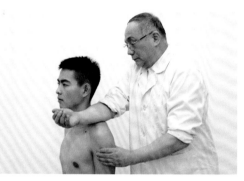

Fig.1-13　Forearm rolling manipulation Ⅴ

Cautions

Manipulator should rotate the forearm in coordination with the flexion and extension of the wrist. Lower the shoulder and drop the elbow to fix on the affected area. Do not lift the elbow and stay close to the skin. This helps to avoid rubbing the body surface which may damage the skin. Manipulator should pay close attention to the patient's posture and use gravity from the upper body swiftly. When performing rolling manipulation, the force used should be increased gradually. Brute force is strictly prohibited to avoid rib fracture or thoracolumbar vertebral fracture.

1.3　Vibrating manipulation

Vibrating manipulation refers to fingers or palms (overlapping palms on the affected area), with continuous and fast vibration, exerting force on the target area. The vibration can be horizontal as well as vertical. Or place the middle finger on the treatment area, with the thumb and index finger against the end of the unbent middle finger. Use this method for continuous and rapid vertical vibration.

Treatment requirements

It is necessary to be as close as possible to the skin, and apply a high frequency vibration, of about 250 times per minute. The force should penetrate deeply. Vibration should only come from the shoulders, arms and hands, while the performer's whole body keeps steady. When performing the "Needle-finger vibrating manipulation", the middle finger should stay on the affected area without lifting to vibrate the patient's skin without damaged. (Fig.1-14; Fig.1-15)

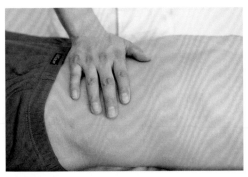

Fig.1-14　Vibrating manipulation on the abdomen

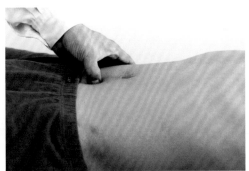

Fig.1-15　Needle-finger vibrating manipulation

The main applicable regions

Points in the abdomen, such as *ShenQue*(CV8), *Qihai*(CV6), *Xiawan*(CV10), *Zhongwan* (CV12), *Shangwan*(CV13). And the points on the head, *Baihui*(GV20), *Fengchi*(GB20), *Yifeng*(SJ17), are also included. The *Baliao*(BL31, BL32, BL33, BL34) lumbosacral points are used sometimes as well.

Cautions

The practitioner's hands cannot leave the affected area and pressing too hard is also forbidden. Instead, use the aid of vibration to penetrate subtly. Practitioner needs to breathe naturally, stand with feet parallel apart and the soles of the feet griping the ground. The tongue should be pressed against the palate to be concentrate and direct strength to the hands. 250 vibrations per minute is best for transferring energy to deep locations. Before treating patients, books, windows or doors can be used for practice. This type of training helps us have a better understanding of the strength of the hands. Later on, the practice can be performed on pillows and quilts to improve the sensitivity of the hands. Finally, hanging paper can be used to realize the sympathetic connection of the paper and vibrating hands.

1.4　Pointing manipulation

Pointing manipulation refers to pressing the specific points by increasing finger force, instead of applying needles. Its effects include clearing and activating the channels and collaterals, dredging zang and fu and regulating Qi. With this convenient technique, it's easy to control the strength and apply moderate stimulation to all points.(Fig.1-16; Fig.1-17)

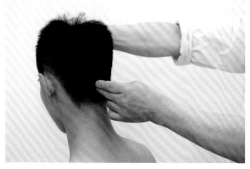

Fig.1-16　Pointing *Yamen*(GV15)

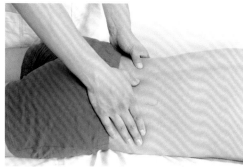

Fig.1-17　Pointing manipulation on the back

Treatment requirements

After placing the fingers on the proper point, gradually increase the strength continuously to stimulate deep tissues.

Cautions

To avoid self damage, keep the proper posture of the fingers at all times. Do not over extend or over bend the fingers.

1.5　Pushing manipulation

Pushing manipulation refers to applying force to certain parts of the human body with fingers, palms, elbows or other parts of body. Make a line or arc shaped movement forward and backward, upward and downward, or leftward and rightward. Pushing manipulation has the effect of clearing and activating the channels and collaterals, removing stagnation, invigorating the circulation of blood and relieving spasms.

Treatment requirements

Apply steady pressure with hand, push slowly, and keep pressure against the affected area. Stay close to the skin, light but not hovering, heavy but not lagging. Follow the directions of channels and blood circulation when performing.

(1) *Pad thumb pushing manipulation*

Apply force with the thumb pad, and the other fingers cling to the other side of the body. Treat the affected part with continuous force from the bending and stretching of the interphalangeal joints, and the swinging of the wrist joints. (Fig.1-18)

(2) *Heel of hand pushing manipulation*

Place the thenars of one hand to the treatment site, fingers stretched, shoulders relaxed, and elbow sunken. Push in one direction with slow, heavy flexion and extension of the elbow joint. Alternate with the other hand. (Fig.1-19)

(3) *Thumb pushing manipulation*

Apply the thumb pads to the affected areas with force and keep the fingers stretched to assist. Follow the route along the channels or parallel to the muscle fiber. (Fig.1-20)

(4) *Elbow pushing manipulation*

Bend your elbow, and push unidirectional with the bulge end of the ulna against the affected areas. (Fig.1-21)

(5) *Outward and inward pushing manipulation*

Performing with both of your hands, pushing away from the central axis to both sides

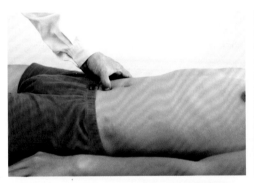
Fig.1-18　Pad thumb pushing manipulation

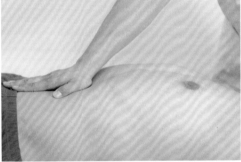
Fig.1-19　Heel of hand pushing manipulation

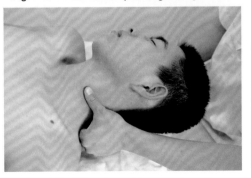
Fig.1-20　Thumb pushing manipulation

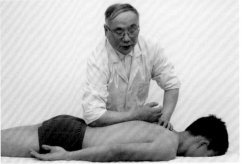
Fig.1-21　Elbow pushing manipulation

of the body is called outward pushing. Pushing from the two sides of the body towards the central axis is called inward pushing, which is commonly used on infants. (Fig.1-22)

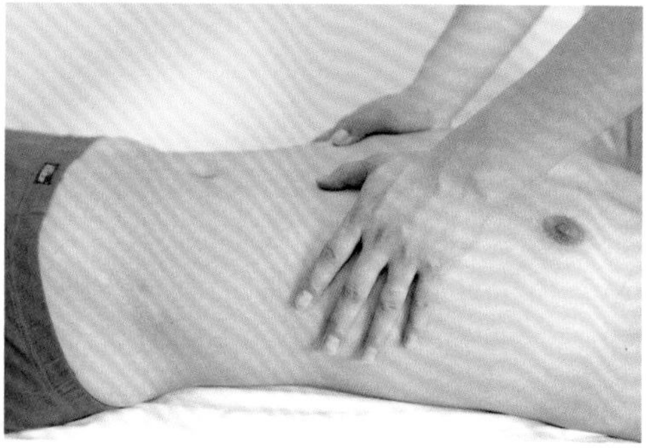

The main applicable regions

Chest, abdomen, extremities, lumbar, back and head.

Cautions

Fig.1-22　Outward and inward pushing manipulation

In the application of this manipulation, the level effected should be deep. Push hard and slow, and do not scratch the skin. All the upper joints work in collaboration to deliver pressure to the treatment area.

1.6　Grasping manipulation

Grasping manipulation is performed by pinching a certain part or point with a clamp formed by the thumb and fingers. The force is generated from the flexion and extension of wrist and finger joints. That is to grasp and lift. Grasping has the effects of clearing and activating the channels and collaterals, relieving spasms and pain, relieving soft tissue adhesion and fatigue.

Treatment requirements

The wrist is relaxed during manipulation, and the fingers are used by keeping the finger joints straight and still. Do not use the plam. Apply force with the finger pads. The lifting direction should be vertical to the muscle. Lift and hold for a moment before releasing the muscle tissue. The force should be smoothly, built up and eased down, no sudden force. This method is the standard for areas with partial swelling and slight pain, or feeling comfortable after release. Pinching and lifting should be continuous and you can move when lifting. Repeat 5 to 10 times.

(1) *Two-finger grasping manipulation*

Apply force with your thumb and index finger. Grasp the skin of the affected area of operation, build up force and pull toward you. Lift the skin, make squeezing and kneading movement with alternating force. (Fig.1-23)

(2) *Three-finger grasping manipulation*

Apply force with your thumb pad, index finger and middle finger. Pinch the skin of the affected area, build up force and grasp toward you. Lift the skin, and make squeezing and kneading movement with alternating force. (Fig.1-24)

(3) *Five-finger grasping manipulation*

Apply force with your thumb and four fingers. Grasp the skin of the affected area and build up force by grasping toward you. Lift the skin, make squeezing and kneading movement with alternating force. (Fig.1-25)

(4) *" 八 " shaped grasping manipulation*

Grasping with both hands towards each other. The hands form the shape of the Chinese character eight (八). Apply force by pushing your hands together, and lifting the affected area. This method is mainly applied to the neck and shoulder. (Fig.1-26)

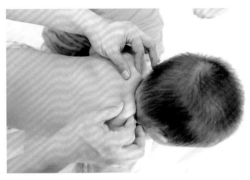

Fig.1-23　Two-finger grasping manipulation

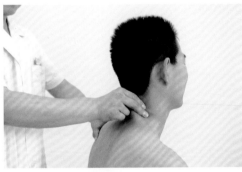

Fig.1-24　Three-finger grasping manipulation

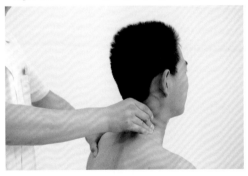

Fig.1-25　Five-finger grasping manipulation

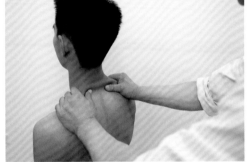

Fig.1-26　"八" shaped grasping manipulation

The main applicable regions

Neck, shoulders, limbs.

Cautions

The grasping manipulation stimulation should be strong. The fingers should be extended and contact the skin with the finger pads like a clamp. Finger joints should be straight. Do not apply force with the sharp fingertips in order to avoid causing discomfort.

1.7 Pressing manipulation

Pressing manipulation is applied by increasing pressure with your palm, elbow or other parts to the affected area. Pressing manipulation has the effect of clearing tendons and veins, relieving spasms and regulating disorders of small joints.

Treatment requirements

Press vertically while varying the force from light to heavy steady and continuous. Use the force to reach the proper depth of the tissue.

(1) *Palm pressing manipulation*

While keeping your wrist back, apply vertical pressure downward with the heel of your hand or the whole palm against the affected area. Use single or both palms. This manipulation is often used alongside others, for example, combined with kneading as pressing kneading and rubbing as pressing rubbing. (Fig.1-27)

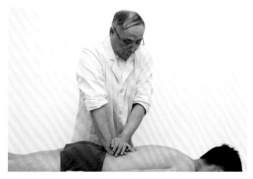

Fig.1-27　Palm pressing manipulation

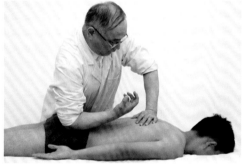

Fig.1-28　Elbow pressing manipulation

(2) *Elbow pressing manipulation*

The manipulator bends his elbow and presses with the end of his elbow, along with some kneading and plucking. This manipulation has a stronger simulating effect. And it is applicable to areas of soft tissue deep in the body. (Fig.1-28)

(3) *Thumb pressing manipulation*

With the thumb straight, use the tip or pad on the affected area. Press down vertically with the help of the four fingers. (Fig.1-29)

(4) *Back pressing manipulation*

Start with both palms against the center of

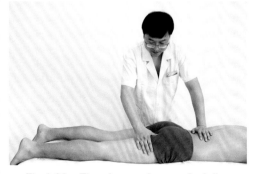

Fig.1-29　Thumb pressing manipulation

the back. Tell the patient to inhale deeply, and exhale deeply. At the end of the exhale, the manipulator's hands press down at the same time, and apply a sudden force. A successful reset is indicated by a snap sound. (Fig.1-30)

(5) *Cross over pressing manipulation*

(Spinous process dislocated to the left as the case) With the patient in the prone position, the manipulator stands at the patient's left side. Places the heel of the left hand to the near the right side of the spine. The heel of the right hand goes to the left side of the spine and slightly away from it. Cross the hands over each other. Apply a sudden downward force at the end of the exhale with more pressure on the right hand. A successful reset is indicated by a snap sound. (Fig.1-31)

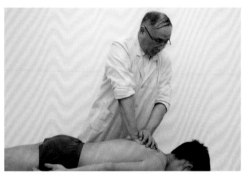 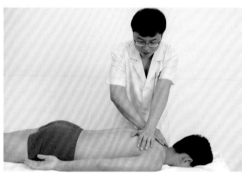

Fig.1-30　Back pressing manipulation　　Fig.1-31　Cross over pressing manipulation

Cautions

In the application of this manipulation, select the focusing point according to the treatment area. When operating on the back, never apply force when the patient is inhaling, at the end of inhaling or exhaling, otherwise you may cause harm to the patient.

1.8　Kneading and twisting manipulation

Kneading and twisting is achieved by making soft and slow circular movements against certain areas or points with your thenar, heel of hand or finger pad. *Bao Chi Tui Na Fa* says, kneading is pressing the points with fingers and making circular movements. *Li Zheng An Mo Yao Shu* says, kneading is diverted from rubbing, make soft slow circular movements with your hand. The force should be light and slow. The effected level should be the subcutaneous tissues, or reach deeper into the muscle. The effect is to relieve spasms and eliminate fatigue. In addition, it can produce an effect of regulating gastrointestinal functions when it is applied to the abdomen.

Treatment requirements

During manipulation, make small scale circular movements with the distal ends of your limbs driven by the proximal ends. Fingers or palm should remain on the skin and make the subcutaneous tissue slide underneath. Apply pressure evenly and move with rhythm. When manipulating, all joints must be relaxed. Drive the wrist with your shoulder and elbow.

(1) *Thumb kneading manipulation*

Make a soft and slow circular movements against certain areas or points with your finger pads. The affected area is small, and the force should be deep and steady. (Fig.1-32)

(2) *Heel of hand kneading manipulation*

With the wrist slightly bend backward, thumb and fingers relaxed, apply force from the heel of your hand. Bend the elbow joint to 160°, shoulder joints down naturally, and wrist joint relaxed. Apply force from the circular movement of aforementioned joints to the area of treatment. The effect area is large, and the stimulation is mild and comfortable. (Fig.1-33)

(3) *Palm kneading manipulation*

Similar to heel of hand kneading, make soft and slow circular movement against certain areas with your palm. (Fig.1-34)

(4) *Thenar kneading manipulation*

Similar to heel of hand kneading, make soft and slow circular movements against certain

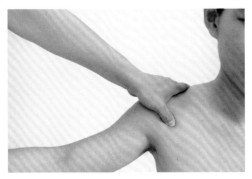

Fig.1-32　Thumb kneading manipulation

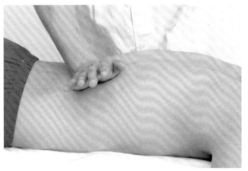

Fig.1-33　Heel of hand kneading manipulation

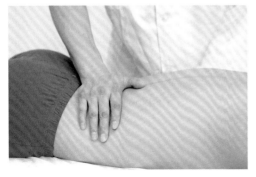

Fig.1-34　Palm kneading manipulation

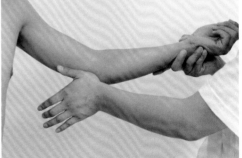

Fig.1-35　Thenar kneading manipulation

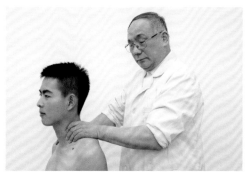

Fig.1-36   Four fingers point-kneading
manipulation

areas or point with your thenars. (Fig.1-35) (5) *Four fingers point-kneading manipulation* Place four fingers (index, middle, ring, and little finger) to the area of treatment, close to each other and slightly bent. Clinch to the skin, and place thumb to the other side of the body or relaxed. Apply continuous force from the circular movement of upper arm and flexion and extension of the wrist. Often used along with four fingers plucking. Commonly used for both sides of the cervical spine muscle groups. (Fig.1-36)

The main applicable regions

Lumbar, chest and abdomen, limbs, head and face.

Cautions

In the application of this manipulation, finger and wrist joints should be relaxed, and never carve or nip the area of treatment. Note: when clinching to the area of treatment and applying force, it's important to use the proper scale of movement. Either too larger or too small will prohibit relaxation. When being applied to the waist, back and extremities, the force should be deep enough to reach the muscle. When being applied to the abdomen, press into the stomach and intestine to create the sour and numb feeling, and distending pain. When being applied to a point, in practice, manipulator often uses combined manipulations like pressing and vibrating.

1.9   Circular rubbing manipulation

Place the finger surface or palm touching on the affected area and make rhythmic and circular movements. This manipulation is called circular rubbing manipulation. The manipulation is soft and the force is moderate on the body surface. Its effects include regulating qi to soothe the chest, soothing the liver to harmonize the stomach, promoting digestion to remove food stagnation, activating blood and resolving stasis, regulating the stomach and intestine functions.

Treatment requirements

With a slightly flexed elbow, relaxed wrist and upper limb, touch the affected area with the palm naturally. Make an active movement of the forearm to create circular rubbing with the palm and wrist. The frequency is 100 times per minute in either a clockwise or counterclockwise direction. The force should be light not too heavy and the frequency should be slow and even. (Fig.1-37)

The main applicable regions

Head, face, chest and abdomen.

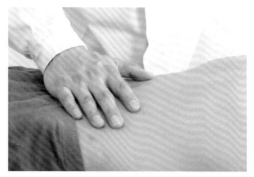

Fig.1-37   Circular rubbing manipulation

1.10   Sweeping manipulation

Place the heel of the palm touching the affected area. Push the wrist forward with the hand and sway left and right. This manipulation is called sweeping manipulation. Its effects include relaxing the muscles and activating the blood circulation, dissipating stasis to subdue swelling, relieving spasm and stopping pain. It is usually used together with pushing manipulation.

Treatment requirements

While performing this manipulation, the palm should be closely attached to the scalp with mild force to avoid rubbing on the skin. The speed should be gradually pushing forward from slow to quick. Repeat the manipulation several times. (Fig.1-38)

Note: Clearing and dissipating manipulation

The doctor gently supports the patient's head with one hand. With the other hand touch the patient's temporal region with the radial side of the thumb and tips of the other fingers.

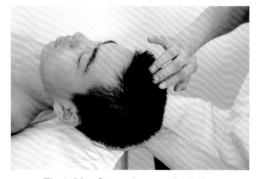

Fig.1-38   Sweeping manipulation

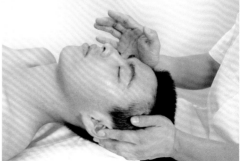

Fig.1-39   Clearing and dissipating manipulation

Push and scrub the hand back and forth. This manipulation has the effect of regulating the qi from *shaoyang*, therefore it is often used to treat diseases as headache, dizziness and hypertension. This manipulation is applied on both side of the head. (Fig.1-39)

Treatment requirements

While performing this manipulation, the force should be light and not heavy. The affected level is just under the skin. The patient will feel relaxed after the treatment.

Cautions

While performing this manipulation, the movement should be done forward and backward along meridians.

1.11 Rotating manipulation

Rotating manipulation refers to those movements in which the manipulator rotates the patient's injured joints slowly and gently. Its effects include relaxing the muscles and activating the blood circulation, releasing adhesions, and improving the amplitude of joint movement, etc.

Treatment requirements

Choose corresponding manipulation according to the different joints. The manipulator usually takes one hand to stabilize the proximal part of the joint and the other hand to hold the distal part, then rotates the joint with steady and gentle force. The force should increase gradually. According to the physiological and pathological joint range of motion, the rotation range should be varied from narrow to broad. It is allowed to exceed the pathological limit, but it should not exceed the physiological limit. Rotate according to the limit patient can stand or doctor's experience. This manipulation is also used

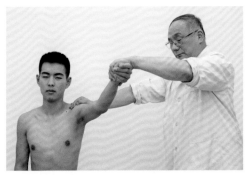

Fig.1-40　Rotating manipulation Ⅰ

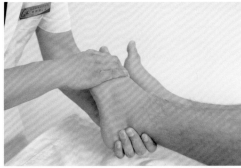

Fig.1-41　Rotating manipulation Ⅱ

together with pulling manipulation. Rotating manipulation used on each part of the body is described in the second chapter. (Fig.1-40 to Fig.1-42)

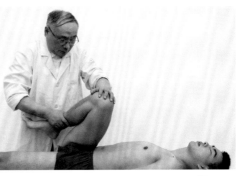

The main applicable regions

Neck and nape, shoulder, elbow, wrist, fingers, lumber, knee, hip and ankle.

Cautions

Fig.1-42　Rotating manipulation Ⅲ

The movement of neck-rotating manipulation should be moderate and mild with steady force. The frequency of rotation should be slow and even. Patient should keep the eyes open to avoid dizziness. It is forbidden to be used to treat patients with fracture. And for the patient with joint function disturbance caused by fracture sequelae, this manipulation should be used with caution to avoid another fracture.

1.12　Shaking manipulation

The shaking manipulation uses one hand or both hands to hold the distal part of the patient's affected limbs and shake it with small amplitude and continuous upward and downward movement. Shaking has the effects of clearing the main and collateral channels, and smoothing the joints. Commonly used to treat injury, adhesion and function disorder of muscle and joints in limbs.

Treatment requirements

The manipulator should hold the distal end of the affected limb, and make shake with force from the wrist. The force should be firm and continuous. The rhythm from slow to fast. The shaking amplitude should be small. Apply stretching force to let the shaking force transmit to the proximal end joint of the extremity.

(1) *The shoulder shaking manipulation*

The patient should be seated. The manipulator should stand at the patient's side and hold the wrist or palm of the affected limb. Then lift it by a 70° -80° angle to the shoulder and pull first. While pulling, shake continuously with a small amplitude. Use an even and fast upward and downward shaking movement.

The purpose is to let the vibration transmit from the wrist to the shoulder where the joints shake most intensely. In the process, you can instantly increase shaking scale 3-5 times. But only intensify the shaking scale, not the pulling force. (Fig.1-43)

(2) *The hip shaking manipulation*

The patient should take the supine position, and the manipulator stand by the patient's feet, then hold the patient's ankle and lift the affected limb off the bed by about 30cm. Pull first, and while pulling, make continuous, fast, upward and downward shaking movements. Apply more force but less frequency than that of the upper limbs. (Fig.1-44)

(3) *The lumbar shaking manipulation*

The patient should take prone position. An assistant may be present to secure the patient by the armpit. The patient may secure him/her self by holding the both edges of the bed. The manipulator should hold up both of the patient's ankles by a small angle and keep his own arms straight. Apply opposite force together with the assistant and stretch the patient's lumbar by leaning backward. When the patient's lumbar is relaxed, the manipulator, while keeping his position, should lean forward first, and then backward. Apply a sudden force and shake upward and downward. Focus most of the shaking effect to the lumbar area. (Fig.1-45; Fig.1-46)

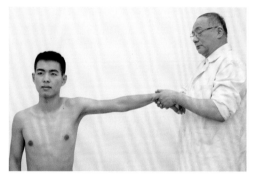

Fig.1-43   The shoulder shaking manipulation

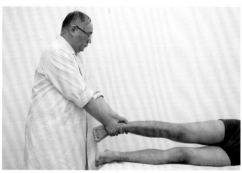

Fig.1-44   The hip shaking manipulation

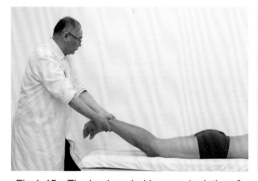

Fig.1-45   The lumbar shaking manipulation Ⅰ

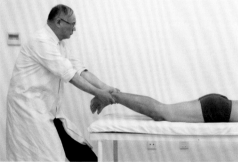

Fig.1-46   The lumbar shaking manipulation Ⅱ

1.13 Concentrating manipulation

Putting two hands or two thumbs on the opposite locations of the affected area to squeeze to the center. This is called concentrating manipulation. Its effects include removing stasis and relaxing tendons to stop pain. (Fig.1-47)

Treatment requirements

When performing the concentrating manipulation, both palms or thumbs should squeeze the affected area with lifting up force. Concentrating also works sliding along the surface of the limbs.

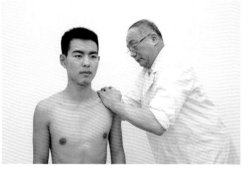

Fig.1-47　Concentrating manipulation

The main applicable regions

Neck and shoulder.

Cautions

Force generated from both hands should be coordinated to make a good tautness, so as to make the patient feel relaxed and comfortable. It is often used as a finishing manipulation.

1.14　Pinching manipulation

The pinching manipulation refers to the manipulator holds the patient's skin and some subcutaneous tissues and pulls them up with the thumb and other fingers. It is often applied to the bilateral sides of an infant's spine. This is called spine pinching. Spine pinching manipulation is not only commonly used for treating children, but also used for treating adults. This manipulation can regulate the functions of organs and is especially good for regulating the functions of stomach and intestines. It can strengthen the body resistance and also has effect on treating insomnia. The movement is manipulated upward along the spine from the natal cleft to the point *Dazhui*(GV14). Repeat the whole manipulation 3 to 5 times until the skin becomes slightly red. On the last time repetition, the manipulator should lift once for every three pinching manipulations. This is called lifting once for every three pinches. The purpose is to increase the stimulation. The pinching manipulation can not only works on the governor vessel, but also works on the bladder meridian of foot-*taiyang*.

Treatment requirements

When pinching forward, the manipulation should be performed continuously and in a straight line without deflection. It should be one lift for every three pinches and repeated for 3 to 5 times. For children, the manipulation is done rhythmically with mild and even force. The movements should be soft and dexterous.

(1) *Three-finger pinching manipulation*

The infant patient takes a prone position. With the wrist in dorsiflexion support the skin of the bilateral sides of the spine with the thumb. Press forward with the index and middle finger; then pinch and lift the skin with three fingers simultaneously with opposite force; perform the lifting and pinching manipulations with both hands alternately and move forward.(Fig.1-48)

(2) *Two-finger pinching manipulation*

The infant patient takes a prone position. With the wrist flexed towards the ulnar, the manipulator uses the radial aspect of the middle knuckle of the flexed index finger. Touch the infant's skin of the bilateral sides of the spine, then moves the thumb forward so as to press the skin. Pinch it with the thumb and index finger. The manipulator performs the lifting and pinching manipulations with both hands alternately and moving forward from the point *Guiwei*(GV1) to the point *Dazhui*(GV14).(Fig.1-49)

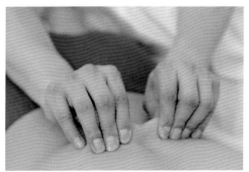

Fig.1-48　Three-finger pinching manipulation　　Fig.1-49　Two-finger pinching manipulation

The main applicable regions

Governor vessel and the bladder meridian of foot-*taiyang*.

Cautions

Pinching steadily with coordination between both hands. The manipulation should be performed in a straight line without deflection with mild and even force. The force of manipulation should be regulated according to patient's disease type deficiency or excess. Dexterous and soft manipulation means reinforcing method. Strong stimulation pulling, grasping, lifting and pinching are reducing methods.

1.15 Knocking manipulation

Knocking manipulation refers to treating the affected area by knocking it with fist, finger, or back of your hand. It has the effect of limbering up muscle and bones, relieving spasms and stopping pain, dispelling fatigue. This manipulation is often used to treat muscle pain, spasm or as follow up treatment after the manipulations with strong stimulation.

Treatment requirements

This manipulation is vigorous and it has a strong simulating effect. So, the manipulation should be skillful when performing. Use one hand or both hands alternately, be relaxed and natural and do not hesitate, be firm and gentle with no hesitation.

(1) *The palm beating manipulation*

With fingers and thumb close to each other, bend your wrist backward and knock the affected area with rhythm. (Fig.1-50)

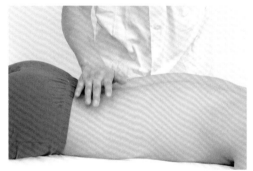

Fig.1-50　The palm beating manipulation　　Fig.1-51　The ulnar side knocking manipulation

(2) *The ulnar side knocking manipulation*

Knocking the affected area with both ulnar of your hands rhythmically and alternately. (Fig.1-51)

(3) *The Fingertip knocking manipulation*

With all thumbs and fingers slightly bent and forming a halfway fist. The fingers are slightly relaxed to retain some flexibility. Wrists are relaxed so they can be driven to sway by the flexion and extension of the elbow joints. Knock the affected area rhythmically with your fingertips. (Fig.1-52)

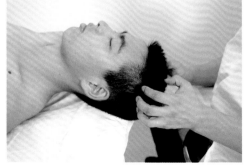

Fig.1-52　The Fingertip knocking manipulation

The palm and ulnar side knocking manipulation have the effect of relieving muscular spasms and eliminating muscle fatigue through vibration. The fingertip knocking manipulation has the effect of inducing resuscitation and refreshment, and improving head blood circulation.

The main applicable regions

- The palm knocking manipulation: lumbosacral region and lower limbs.
- The ulnar side knocking manipulation: neck and shoulder, the four limbs.
- The fingertip knocking manipulation: head.

Cautions

There should be a certain rhythmic while performing so that the patient would feel relaxed and comfortable. It is often used as a finishing manipulation.

1.16   Palm-twisting manipulation

Palm-twisting manipulation refers to grip a certain part of the extremity with both palms. Perform swiftly twisting and kneading to and fro movement with opposite force.

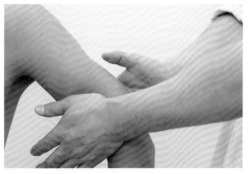

The movement is coupled with a vertical motion. Its effects include dredging the meridians, regulating qi and blood, and relaxing muscles. The manipulation is often used to treat soft tissue injuries, muscle and tendon spasm and pain. It's also used after strong stimulating manipulations. (Fig.1-53)

Fig.1-53   Palm-twisting manipulation

Treatment requirements

The force used by both hands should be balanced. The manipulation demands rapid twisting and slow moving. The affected tissue layer should be from the deeper to the superficial. This manipulation is often used as a final manipulation.

The main applicable regions

The upper limbs.

Cautions

The force should be steady and the moving action should be slow.

1.17　Patting manipulation

The patting manipulation refers to slightly patting on the affected area with the palm driven by the wrist and elbow joints. The patting manipulation has the effect of relieving tendons and smoothing collaterals and improving the blood circulations. This manipulation can be used for the treatment of shoulder and back pain, dysmenorrhea, skelalgia and sour smelling feet. Besides, patting on the back also has the effect of resolving phlegm and relieving cough. (Fig.1-54)

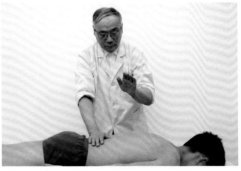

Fig.1-54　Patting manipulation

Treatment requirements

Keep fingers closed together and slightly bent, with the wrist relaxed, wave your forearms to drive the wrist joints swaying freely. Fingers land first and wrist next. Wrist lifts first and fingers next. Beat the body surface with full palms. The force should be proper and make a small sweeping movement when landing wrists in order to intensify the effect of the force.

The main applicable regions

Shoulder, back and lumbosacral region. You can also pat top-down along the gallbladder meridians of foot-*shaoyang* at both sides of the thighs.

Cautions

Professor Cui's clinical applications of patting manipulation makes use of the full palms, which is different from those using half palm recorded in common books. His theory is that full palms are easier to convey the force and help to relax the wrist. And after gaining some experience, make a small sweeping movement when landing wrists to deliver a better relaxing effect. The force should be proper and not to cause pain to the patient, and pat rhythmically.

1.18　Linear rubbing manipulation

Place the palm on the treatment area. Make an active movement of the upper arm to create a to and fro straight line rubbing movement. The direction can be up and down or left and right. This manipulation is called linear rubbing manipulation. It can worm the meridians, promote qi and activate blood. It is often used to treat cold type disease. The heat effect induced by rubbing can penetrate into the deep layers through the body surface and make the patient will feel warm. This is called "penetrating warm". This manipulation is often used as a final manipulation.

Treatment requirements

The rubbing movement should go to and fro along a straight line without deflection. The palm should be kept close to the affected area. The pressing force should be moderate. The movement must be continous without halting. The frequency should be kept even and fast.

(1) *Linear rubbing manipulation with palm*

Place the palm close to the affected areas Move the upper arm intuitively with the palm rubbing on the body surface to and fro along a straight line. In this manipulation, the contact area is larger so there is less heat produced. It is often applied on back, lumbar region, and shoulder. (Fig.1-55)

(2) *Linear rubbing manipulation with hypothenar*

Place the hypothenar close to the affected area. Move the upper arm intuitively with the hypothenar rubbing on the body surface to and fro along a straight line. In this manipulation, the contact area is smaller. So that with the same pressure to the skin, more friction heat can be generated more and quicker. It is often applied on lumbosacral region, shoulder and back, extremities. (Fig.1-56)

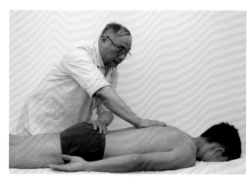
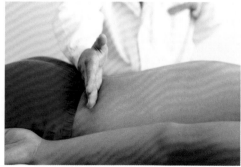

Fig.1-55   Linear rubbing manipulation with palm

Fig.1-56   Linear rubbing manipulation with hypothenar

Cautions

The treatment area should be exposed. Lubricant, such as massage lotion or turpentine oil is often used on affected area.

Chapter 2

Tuina Manipulations Applied on Different Part of the Body

2.1 Tuina manipulations applied on the head

2.1.1 Basic tuina manipulations applied on the head

The basic tuina manipulations applied on the head mainly refers to "Cui's ten tuina manipulations used on the head". The principles of treatment are dredging meridians, unblocking collaterals, circulating qi and blood and reducing pain. Patient with external disease factors should be stimulated seriously into a sweat while the patient with internal injuries should be stimulated softly to reduce the pain. During the treatment, perform the manipulation slowly, softly and evenly, the force should be from light to heavy, and then from heavy to light. The feelings of comfort, numbness and distension is normal for the patient.

Posture selection:

Ask the patient to adopt a supine posture and the manipulator sits in front of patient's head.

(1) *Opening Tianmen(heaven gate)*

The line from the midpoint *Yintang*(EX-HN3) between the two eyebrows to the anterior hairline *Shengting*(GV24). Push from the point straight upward with the pads of both thumbs alternately. Repeat the manipulation 3 to 5 times.(Fig.2-1)

(2) *Pressing three meridians*

Press on the three lines from *Yintang*(EX-HN3) to *Baihui*(GV20), from *Yuyao*(EX-HN4) to *Sishencong*(EX-HN1) and from

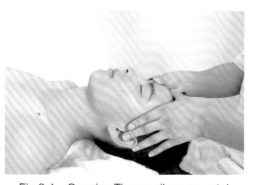

Fig.2-1 Opening Tianmen(heaven gate)

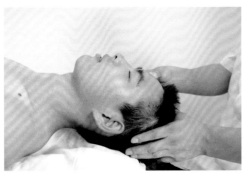

Fig.2-2　Pressing three meridians Ⅰ

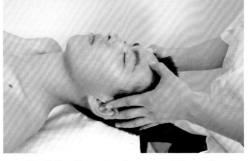

Fig.2-3　Pressing three meridians Ⅱ

Shuaigu(GB8) to *Baihui*(GV20) straight upward with both thumbs.(Fig.2-2 to Fig.2-4)

(3) *Separating yin and yang*

Push from a point separating outwards to both side or from the middle line of forehead to both sides respectively with the pads of both thumbs. Repeat the manipulation 3 to 5 times. (Fig.2-5)

(4) *Scraping the eyebrow arc*

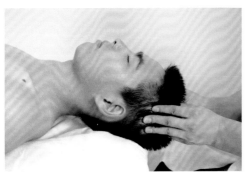

Fig.2-4　Pressing three meridians Ⅲ

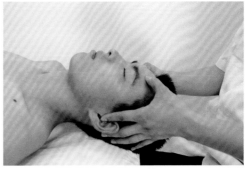

Fig.2-5　Separating yin and yang

Scrape the line respectively from the medial ends of the eyebrows *Cuanzhu*(BL2) to the lateral ends *Sizhukong*(TE23) with both thumbs. Repeat the manipulation for 2 minutes. (Fig.2-6)

(5) *Pressing points following meridians*

Press the following points one by one along the meridians for 5 to 10 times. The points are *Jingming*(BL1), *Cuanzhu* (BL2), *Yuyao*(EX-HN4), *Sizhukong*(TE23), *Chengqi*(ST1), *Sibai*(ST2), *Yingxiang* (LI20), *Jiache*(ST6), *Dicang*(ST4),

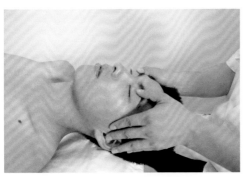

Fig.2-6　Scraping the eyebrow arc

Chengjiang(CV24), *Jinjin*(EX-HN12), *Yuye*(EX-HN13), *Yifeng*(TE17), *Touwei*(ST8), *Baihui*(GV20), *Wangu*(GB12), *Shuaigu*(GB8), *Fengchi*(GB20). (Fig.2-7; Fig.2-8; Table 2-1)

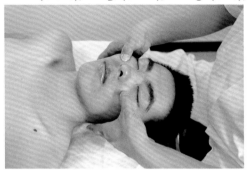
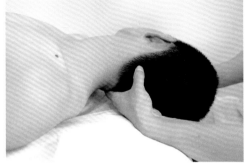

Fig.2-7　Pressing *Sibai*(ST2)　　　　　Fig.2-8　Pressing *Fengchi*(GB20)

Table 2-1　The locations of the points used in "Pressing points following meridians"

Point	Location
Jingming(BL1)	On the face, in the depression slightly above the inner canthus.
Cuanzhu(BL2)	On the face, in the depression of the midial end of the eyebrow, at the supraorbital notch.
Yuyao(EX-HN4)	Directly above the pupils when the eyes are looking straight forwards, in the center of the eyebrow.
Sizhukong(TE23)	In the depression of the lateral end of the eyebrow.
Chengqi(ST1)	On the face, directly below the pupil with the eyes looking straight forward, between the eyeball and the infraorbital ridge.
Sibai(ST2)	On the face, directly below the pupil with the eyes looking straight forward, in the depression of the infraorbital foramen.
Yingxiang(LI20)	0.5 *cun* beside the lateral border of the nasal ala, in the nasolabial groove.
Jiache(ST6)	On the cheek, one finger breadth anterior and superior to the mandibular angle, in the depression where the masseter muscle is prominent.
Dicang(ST4)	On the face, 0.4 *cun* beside the mouth angle.
Chengjiang(CV24)	On the face, in the depression at the midpoint of the mentolabial sulcus.
Jinjin(EX-HN12)	In the mouth, on the two veins under the tongue, with *Jinjin*(EX-HN12) on the left.
Yuye(EX-HN13)	In the mouth, on the two veins under the tongue, with *Yuye*(EX-HN13) on the right.
Yifeng(TE17)	Posterior to the lobe, in the depression between the mastoid process and angle of the mandible.
Touwei(ST8)	On the lateral side of the head, 0.5 *cun* above the anterior hairline at the corner of the forehead.
Baihui(GV20)	On the head, 5 *cun* directly above the midpoint of the anterior hairline, at the midpoint of the line connecting the apexes of the both ears.
Wangu(GB12)	In the depression posterior and inferior to the mastoid process.
Shuaigu(GB8)	1.5 *cun* from the apex of the ear straight into the hairline.
Fengchi(GB20)	On the nape, below the occipital bone, in the depression between the upper ends of the sternocleidomastoid and trapezius muscles.

(6) *Pushing with the heel of palm*

Pushing with the heel of palm focus on the following points. The points are *Yintang*

(GV29), Superciliary arch, *Cuanzhu*(BL2), *Shangxing*(GV23), *Jiache*(ST6), etc. The operation can be done at a frequency of 250-500 times per minutes. (Fig.2-9)

(7) *Grasping the scalp*

Grasp the scalp with the pads of both hands fingers from the middle of the head to both sides. (Fig.2-10)

(8) *Sweeping manipulation to treat wind syndrome of head*

Sweeping manipulation is done with the pad of both hands fingers along the three lines. They are from the point *Shenting*(GV4) to point *Baihui*(GV20) on the governor vessel, point *Quchai*(BL4) to point *Tongtian*(BL7) on the bladder meridian, point *Qubin*(GB7) to point *Touwei*(ST8) on the gallbladder meridian and stomach meridian. The operation can be done for one minute at a frequency of 400-600 times per minutes. (Fig.2-11)

(9) *Tapping the scalp*

Tap the scalp gently with the pads of the five fingers. The movement of the fingertips is created by the shaking of the wrist. The operation can be done at a frequency about 200 times per minutes. (Fig.2-12)

(10) *Blowing the face*

First rub hands until hot, then massage the head and face repeatedly. (Fig.2-13)

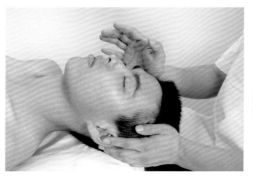

Fig.2-9   Pushing with the heel of palm

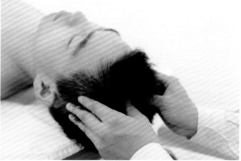

Fig.2-10   Grasping the scalp

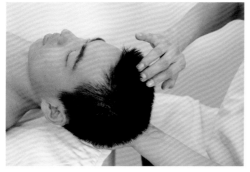

Fig.2-11   Sweeping manipulation to treat wind syndrome of head

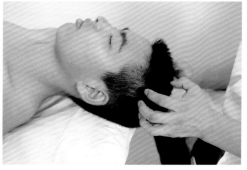

Fig.2-12   Tapping the scalp

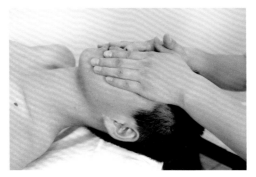

Fig.2-13 Blowing the face

2.1.2 Other tuina manipulations applied on the head

2.1.2.1 The reduction manipulation for temporomandibular joint

Preparation

The patient should sit, back against a wall or the back of a chair. And the level of the patient's inferior dental arch should be lower than the elbow of the doctor. An assistant should be there to fix the patient's head and shoulders to prevent the movement.

Relax the affected area

The doctor should stand in front of the patient. Press and knead the following points *Jiache*(ST6), *Yifeng*(TE17), *Yiming*(EX-HN14), *Shuaigu*(GB8)and *Taiyang*(EX-HN5) for several times to relieve the tension and spasm of the masseter first. Then operate the pointing manipulation on the following points *Jiache*(ST6), *Xiaguan*(ST7), *Ermen*(TE21). And finally, press and knead the point *Hegu*(LI4) on both hands. (Fig.2-14 to Fig.2-17)

Reduction manipulation

Comfort the patient to relax and ask to open the mouth as wide as possible. The doctor should stand in front of the patient, wrapping his thumbs with sterile gauze to avoid being

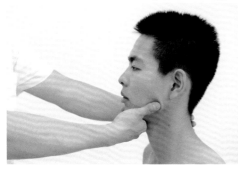

Fig.2-14 Kneading *Jiache*(ST6)

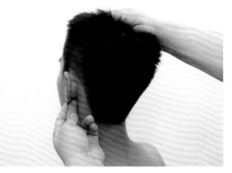

Fig.2-15 Kneading *Yifeng*(TE17)

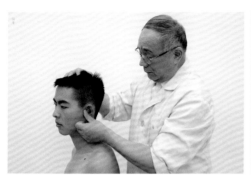

Fig.2-16 Pointing *Ermen*(TE21)

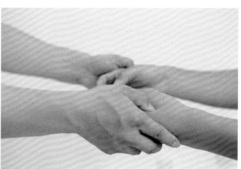

Fig.2-17 Pressing and Kneading
Hegu(LI4) on both hands

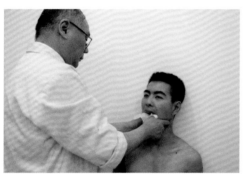

Fig.2-18 The reduction manipulation for
temporomandibular joint

bitten or scratched by teeth. And then put both thumbs into the patient's mouth cavity to fix the inferior dental arch while the other fingers hold the lower jaw. When reducing, press the lower jaw downward with thumbs and pull it outward with the fingers and move the condyloid process down below the articular tubercle, and then push up and inward to send the articular tubercle back to the articular fovea. (Fig.2-18)

After the joint reduction, quickly withdraw thumbs and the sound of articular tubercle sliding back into the articular fossa should be heard or felt. If the manipulation of sending the articular tubercle back to the articular fovea is failed, do not force it, instead, the doctor should further relax the masseter and comfort the patient so as to reach the best treating conditions.

2.1.3 Cases of syndrome differentiation for clinical tuina manipulations

The following diseases should be treated based on the basic tuina manipulations applied first on the head. And then according to the patterns of each syndrome, add or subtract the following manipulations. (Note: Manipulations applied on different parts of the body will be narrated in the following sections)

2.1.3.1 Headache

After operating the "Cui's ten tuina manipulations used on the head" to regulate the qi moving in the meridians, point and knead the pressure points on the face and head. And then, treat based on overall analysis of symptoms and signs.

Commonly used manipulations

Pointing and kneading the following points: *Fengchi*(GB20), *Fengfu*(GV16), *Quchi* (LI11), *Hegu*(LI4), *Waiguan*(TE5), *Zhangmen*(LR13), *Taichong*(LR3), *Xingjian*(LR2), *Cuanzhu*(BL2), *Shenshu*(BL23), *Taixi*(KI3), *Sanyinjiao*(SP6), *Xinshu*(BL15), *Geshu*(BL17), *Pishu*(BL20), *Zusanli*(ST36), *Qihai*(CV6), *Sanjiaoshu*(BL22), *Pishu*(BL20), *Weishu*(BL21), *Gaohuang*(BL43), *Taiyang*(EX-HN5), *Touwei*(ST8), *Zhongwan*(CV12), *Yanglingquan*(GB34), *Fenglong*(ST40). Pushing manipulation on the bladder meridian of foot-*taiyang*. Pushing manipulations on Qiaogong(an oblique line from mastoid process to sternoclavicular joint). Circular-rubbing manipulation on the abdomen. Linear-rubbing manipulation on governor vessel. Grasping manipulation on the lateral sides of the lower limbs. Patting manipulation along the bladder meridian of foot-*taiyang* on the back.

2.1.3.2 Dizziness

In the treatment of dizziness, the four manipulations include "pressing three meridians", "separating yin and yang", "pressing points following meridians" and "blowing the face" are the main treatments from the "Cui's ten tuina manipulations used on the head". And then combine with other manipulations to assist in treating the disease according to differentiation of syndrome.

Commonly used manipulations

Pushing Qiaogong(an oblique line from mastoid process to sternoclavicular joint). Pointing on the following points: *Xinshu*(BL15), *Ganshu*(BL18), *Shenshu*(BL23), *Mingmen*(GV4), *Quchi*(LI11), *Sanyinjiao*(SP6), *Taichong*(LR3). Linear-rubbing manipulation along the bladder meridian of foot-*taiyang* on the back. Scraping the costal arch. Opening four gates (the four gates include four points: *Zhangmen*(LR13), *Qimen*(LR14), *Huaroumen*(ST24), *Riyue*(GB24)). Pointing three wan (the three wan are three points include *Shangwan*(CV13), *Zhongwan*(CV12), *Xiawan*(CV10)). (The upper three manipulations can be seen in section 2.3 Tuina manipulations applied on the thorax and abdomen). Pointing manipulation on the following points: *Baihui*(GV20), *Fengchi*(GB20), *Fengfu*(CV16) and *Yamen*(CV15). Grasping manipulation on the points: *Fengchi*(GB20), *Jianjing*(GB21), *Hegu*(GB4). Tonifying *Shenque*(CV8). Point penetrating *Tianshu*(ST25). Promoting *Qihai*(CV6). (The upper three manipulations can be seen in section 2.3 Tuina manipulations applied on the thorax and abdomen)

2.1.3.3 Insomnia

In the treatment of insomnia, the "Cui's ten tuina manipulations used on the head" is used mainly to dredge the channels, communicate yin and yang of the body. When operating the manipulations, it should be gentle and soft so that the patient will not feel pain. To treat insomnia, before we operate the "Cui's ten tuina manipulations used on the head", we combine with the "Cui's six tuina manipulations used on the back"(it can be seen in section 2.4 Tuina manipulations applied on the back and waist). And then combine these with other manipulations to assist in treating the disease according to differentiation of syndrome.

Commonly used manipulations

Kneading the following points: *Zusanli*(ST36), *Sanyinjiao*(SP6), *Shenmen*(HT7), *Tianshu*(ST25). Pushing Qiaogong(an oblique line from mastoid process to sternoclavicular joint). Linear rubbing manipulation on *Yongquan*(KI1). Kneading the following points: *Ganshu*(BL18), *Danshu*(BL19), *Zhangmen*(LR13), *Qimen*(LR14) and *Taichong*(LR3). Pointing and pressing the following points *Shenmen*(HT7), *Neiguan*(PC6), *Fenglong* (ST40), *Zusanli*(ST36), *Zhongwan*(CV12).

2.1.3.4　Facial paralysis

To treat facial paralysis, the "Cui's ten tuina manipulations used on the head" is used first. In the manipulation of "Pressing points following meridians", focus on pressing the following points: *Jinjin*(EX-HN12), *Yuye*(EX-HN13), *Jiache*(ST6), *Yifeng*(TE17), *Fengchi*(GB20). And then combine with other manipulations to assist in treating the disease according to differentiation of syndrome.

Commonly used manipulations

Pointing the following points: *Fenglong*(ST40), *Zusanli*(ST36), *Chengshan*(BL57), *Yanglingquan*(GB34), *Hegu*(LI4), *Quchi*(LI11), *Shaohai*(HT3), *Taichong*(LR3), *Yongquan*(KI1), *Weizhong*(BL40), *Sanyinjiao*(SP6), *Laogong*(PC8), *Jingmen*(GB25), *Zhaohai*(KI6).

2.2　Tuina manipulations applied on the neck

2.2.1　Basic tuina manipulations applied on the neck

2.2.1.1　Sinew-plucking manipulation on seven lines

The patient takes a sitting posture and the manipulator operates the "Plucking manipulation with the thumb" along the meridians on the following five lines. The first line is from point *Fengfu*(GV16) to point *Dazhui*(GV14) on the governor vessel(Fig.2-19).

The second and third line (one on the left and one on the right) is from point *Tianzhu*(BL10) to point *Dazhu*(BL11) along the bladder meridian of foot-*taiyang*(Fig.2-20). The fourth and fifth line (one on the left and one on the right) is from point *Fengchi* (GB20) to point *Jianjing*(GB21) along the gallbladder meridian of foot-*shaoyang*(Fig.2-21). If the muscle on the patient's shoulder is strong and thick, the manipulation can change into the "Forearm rolling manipulation".

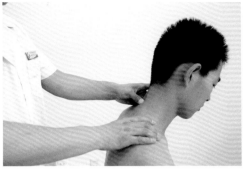

Fig.2-19　Point *Fengfu*(GV16) to point *Dazhui*(GV14)

And then operating the "Plucking manipulation with the four fingers"on the sixth and seventh line (one on the left and one on the right): from point *Yifeng*(TE17) belonging to the triple energizer meridian of hand-*shaoyang* to point *Quepen*(ST12) belonging to the stomach meridian of foot-*yangming*(Fig.2-22; Fig.2-23). There are seven lines in all. The manipulations should be operated on the seven lines from top to bottom, the force should

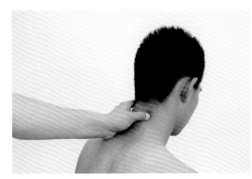

Fig.2-20　Point *Tianzhu*(BL10) to point *Dazhu*(BL11)

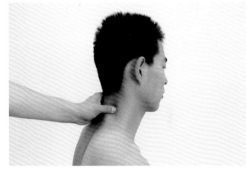

Fig.2-21　Point *Fengchi*(GB20) to point *Jianjing*(GB21)

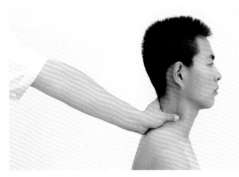

Fig.2-22　Point *Yifeng*(TE17) to point *Quepen*(ST12)

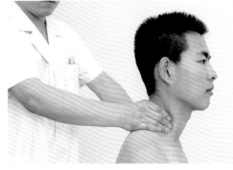

Fig.2-23　Plucking manipulation with the four fingers

from slight to heavy, the position should from middle line to the sides, the normal side should be first followed by the affected side for about 15 minutes. So as to dredge the meridians well rounded and relax the soft tissues on the neck deeply.

2.2.1.2　Rolling manipulation

We can see the rolling manipulation applied on the neck in Fig.2-24, Fig.2-25.

2.2.1.3　Grasping manipulation

We can see the grasping manipulation applied on the neck in Fig.2-26 to Fig.2-28.

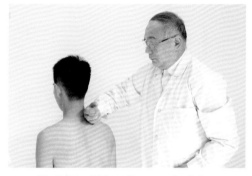

Fig.2-24　Side rolling manipulation

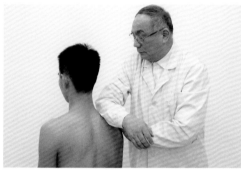

Fig.2-25　Forearm rolling manipulation

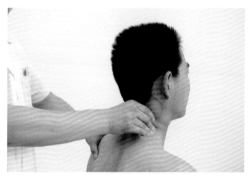

Fig.2-26　Five-fingers grasping manipulation

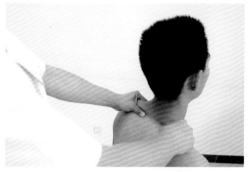

Fig.2-27　"/\" shaped grasping manipulation

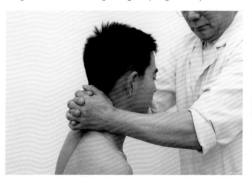

Fig.2-28　Grasping the neck

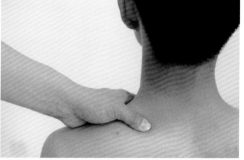

Fig.2-29　Pointing *Jianzhongshu*(SI15)

2.2.1.4 Pointing manipulation

We can see the pointing manipulation applied on the neck in Fig.2-29, Fig.2-30.

2.2.1.5 Lifting manipulation

We can see the lifting manipulation applied on the neck in Fig.2-31, Fig.2-32.

2.2.1.6 Pinching manipulation

We can see the pinching manipulation applied on the neck in Fig.2-33.

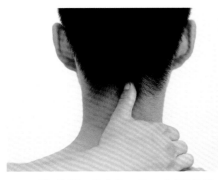

Fig.2-30　Pointing *Fengfu*(GV16)

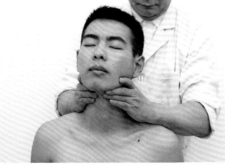

Fig.2-31　Lifting manipulation applied
on neck Ⅰ

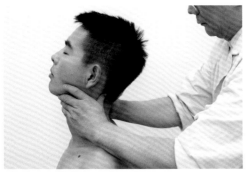

Fig.2-32　Lifting manipulation applied
on neck Ⅱ

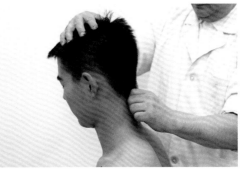

Fig.2-33　Pinching manipulation applied
on the neck

2.2.2　Other tuina manipulations applied on the neck

2.2.2.1 Pushing Qiaogong

Qiaogong is an oblique line from mastoid process (point *Yifeng*(TE17))to sternoclavicular joint(point *Quepen*(ST12)). When operating, apply pushing manipulation from top to bottom with the ventral aspects of the thumb or four fingers. The pressure should be moderate and the skin should not be rubbed. The two sides can not be operated together.

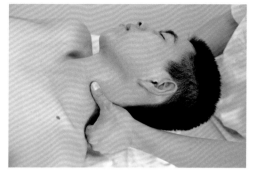

Fig.2-34   Pushing Qiaogong Ⅰ

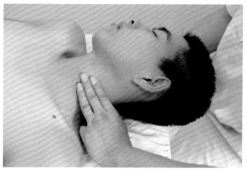

Fig.2-35   Pushing Qiaogong Ⅱ

This manipulation is used to treat hypertension. (Fig.2-34; Fig.2-35)

2.2.2.2   Pulling-extending manipulation with elbow and *Hukou*(the part between the thumb and the four fingers) supporting the neck

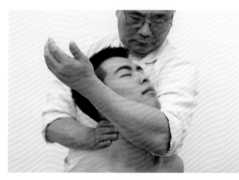

Fig.2-36   Pulling-extending manipulation with elbow and *Hukou*

The patient takes a sitting position with the head leaning and backwards in an extension. The doctor holds the patient's occiput with the part between the thumb and the four fingers of the left hand, holding the patient's chin with the left elbow flexed, rolling it from side to side to relax the joint and then pulling and extending the patient's neck up slowly. (Fig.2-36)

Operational requirements

During performation of the pulling-extending manipulation, the angle of the patient' head backward should be about 30°. Both hands should be fixed on the patient's head steadily and pull with synergy. The pulling-extending can be done after the patient relaxed.

Cautions

According to the illness and patient's condition, decide whether or not the pulling-extending manipulation should be administered. The performance should be done with the strength intensified gradually. The muscles on the neck and shoulder should be relaxed after the manipulation to release muscle tension and reduce pain.

2.2.2.3   Pulling manipulation for locating and rotating cervical vertebrae

Take the left-deflected spinal process of the patient's affected cervical vertebrae for example: the patient takes a sitting position and the doctor stands behind the patient while palpating the deflected spinal process of the cervical vertebrae with both hands.

Press the left side of the spinal process of the patient's affected cervical vertebrae with the right thumb, tell the patient to look down until the deflected spinal process start to move and then tell the patient to bend the head to the opposite side, and rotate the face to the same side of the deflected spinal process to as much as possible. Then the doctor holds the patient's chin with his left hand and waits for the patient relaxed, takes a quick and controlled pulling action along the direction of the rotation within a small increased amplitude. Meanwhile, the right thumb pressing the deflected spinal process pushes and presses towards the opposite side. Cracking sound is often heard if reduction of the joint is successful. (Fig.2-37 to Fig.2-40). The hand holding the chin of patient also can be replaced by the elbow.

Operational requirements

The location should be accurate. The performance should be steady, quick and mild. Turn the joint to the limited degree and then pull steady is a critical step for successful performance of the manipulation.

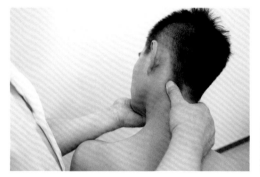

Fig.2-37　Pulling manipulation for locating and rotating cervical vertebrae Ⅰ

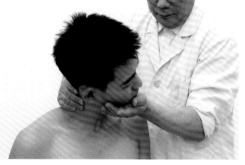

Fig.2-38　Pulling manipulation for locating and rotating cervical vertebrae Ⅱ

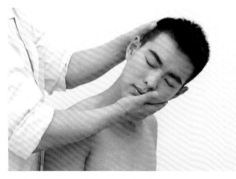

Fig.2-39　Pulling manipulation for locating and rotating cervical vertebrae Ⅲ

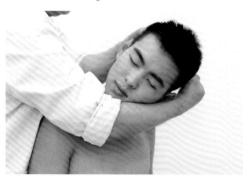

Fig.2-40　Pulling manipulation for locating and rotating cervical vertebrae Ⅳ

Cautions

When operating this manipulation to make the joint reduction on the neck, an inappropriate manipulation might stimulate patient's vertebral artery to make them prostration. In some special situations, a patients may suffer from a iatrogenic spinal cord injury and which may cause serious consequences like the high paraplegic incident. So, when applying this manipulation, the accurate location of the affected cervical vertebrae is the premise to have a good effect. And the doctor's reduction manipulation must be skillful and it is the key to get a better effect. The wrong location, the omitted affected vertebrae, wrong judgment of the direction of the deflected vertebrae should lead to a poor effect or even increase the illness. The location must be accurate, the force should be gentle and soft and violent action should be avoided. Never try to achieve the cracking sound aimlessly. Meanwhile, this manipulation is prohibited to use on advanced patients and the patient who has severe osteoporosis.

2.2.2.4 Manipulation for obliquely-pulling the neck

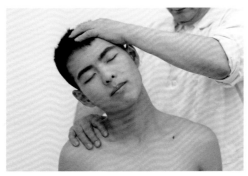

Fig.2-41   Manipulation for obliquely-
pulling the neck

Take the head bending restricted to the left for example: the doctor stands behind the patient, presses the right side of the spinal process of the patient's affected cervical vertebrae with the right hand, holds the left side of the patient's head with the left hand. Ask the patient to bend the cervical vertebrae to the pathological limited degree, until wait for the patient relaxed, and then a quick and controlled rotating pulling is done within a small increased amplitude. Relaxing the hands instantly. (Fig.2-41)

The operational requirements and cautions are basically the same with the "Pulling manipulation for locating and rotating cervical vertebrae".

2.2.2.5 Pointing *Wailaogong*(EX-UE8)

The point *Wailaogong*(EX-UE8) is located on the dorsum of the hand, between the second and third metacarpal bones, 0.5cm posterior to the metacarpo-phalangeal joint.

The patient takes a sitting position. The doctor stands beside the affected side of the patient, tells the patient to lateral raise up the arm laterally on the affected side with the dorsum of the hand upwards. The doctor holds the patient's palm with one hand, and the other hand points the point *Wailaogong*(EX-UE8). Meanwhile, tell the patient to turn his/her head to the affected side slowly to the maximum limit and then turn back to the other direction to the maximum limit. After that, tell the patient to turn his/her head to face forward. Pointing the *Wailaogong*(EX-UE8) on the affected side first and then pointing it on the normal side. During the pointing manipulation, combine with the "Needle-finger vibrating manipulation" will get a better effect. (Fig.2-42)

This manipulation should belong to section: "Tuina manipulations applied on the wrist

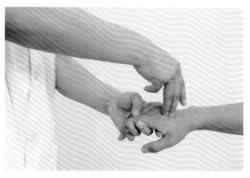

Fig.2-42　Pointing *Wailaogong*(EX-UE8)

and palm" according to the parts of the body. It is because of this manipulation is often used to treat cervical disease so as to classified it into the "Tuina manipulations applied on the neck".

2.2.3　Cases of syndrome differentiation for clinical tuina manipulations

The following diseases should be treated based on the basic tuina manipulations applied on the head first. And then according to the patterns of syndrome,add or subtract the following manipulations.(Attention: Manipulations applied on the other part of the body will be narrated in the following sections)

2.2.3.1　Cervical spondylopathy

The "Sinew-plucking manipulation on seven lines" should be operated first to relax the muscles for 15 minutes. For the patient with cervical spondylotic radiculopathy, pointing and pressing the following points: *Jiquan*(HT1), *Jianzhen*(SI9), *Jianjing*(GB21), *Quepen*(ST12) on the affected side; For the patient with vertebral artery type of cervical spondylosis, pointing and pressing the following points include: *Yamen*(GV15), *Baihui*(GV20), *Yintang*(GV21), *Shangxing*(GV23), *Yifeng*(TE17), *Fengchi*(GB20), *Hegu*(LI4), *Neiguan*(PC6), *Quchi*(LI11), *Shaohai*(HT3) on both sides. The patient with joint malposition, the joint reduction manipulation can be used.

2.2.3.2　Thoracic outlet syndrome

The "Catapult-plucking manipulation"can be used to pluck the anterior and medial scalenus, sternocleidomastoid and their spaces(from point *Yifeng*(TE17) to point *Quepen*(ST12)) for 3-5 minutes. Apply kneading manipulation, plucking manipulation and rolling manipulation on the muscles along the shoulder girdle. Besides, pointing and pressing the points include *Jianjing*(GB21), *Tianzong*(SI11), *Jianwaishu*(SI12), etc. Rotating the upper limb of the affected side for 8-10 times, and after that, pointing and pressing the points include

Jiquan(HT1), *Quchi*(LI11), *Quze*(LU5), *Shousanli*(LI10) and *Hegu*(LI4), etc.

2.2.3.3 Stiff neck

The patient takes a sitting position. The doctor stands behind the patient close to the affected side. Operating the "Thumb kneading manipulation" on the affected area gently and softly to relax the spasmodic muscles. After that, pointing the point *Wailaogong*(EX-UE8).

2.2.3.4 Neck-originated hypertension

Perform the "Cui's ten tuina manipulations used on the head" first, and then the "Cui's six tuina manipulations used on the back" (it can be seen in section 2.4 Tuina manipulations applied on the back and waist), the "Sinew-plucking manipulation on seven lines". After that, combine with other manipulations to assist treating the disease according to differentiation of syndrome.

2.3 Tuina manipulations applied on the thoracic and abdominal region

2.3.1 Basic tuina manipulations applied on the thoracic and abdominal region

2.3.1.1 The Cui's eight tuina manipulations used on the abdomen

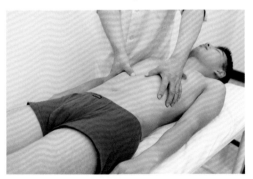

Figf. 2-43   Scraping the costal arch Ⅰ

(1) *Scraping the costal arch*

With both hands thumb pulp to press both sides of the chest, operating the circular rubbing manipulation along the rib 9 to rib 12 for 5 to 10 times. (Fig.2-43 to Fig.2-45)

(2) *Opening four gates* (the four gates are four points including *Zhangmen*(LR13), *Qimen*(LR14), *Huaroumen*(ST24), *Riyue* (GB24))

Performing the thumb pointing manipulation on the following points: *Zhangmen*(LR13), *Qimen*(LR14), *Huaroumen*(ST24), *Riyue*(GB24) for 5 to 10 times. And each point should be pointed 5 to 10 seconds. (Fig.2-46 to Fig.2-49)

(3) *Pointing three wan* (the three wan are three points including *Shangwan*(CV13), *Zhongwan* (CV12), *Xiawan*(CV10))

Performing the "Whorl side thumb pushing manipulation" combine with pointing

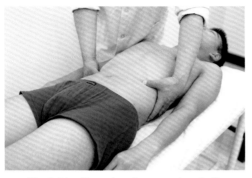

Fig.2-44　Scraping the costal arch II

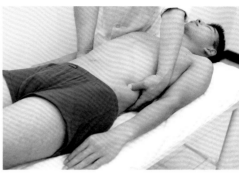

Fig.2-45　Scraping the costal arch III

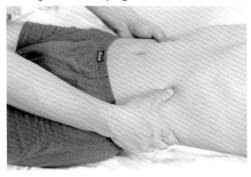

Fig.2-46　Opening four gates-*Zhangmen*(LR13)

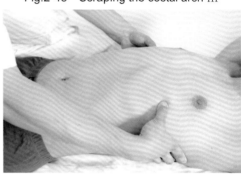

Fig.2-47　Opening four gates-*Qimen*(LR14)

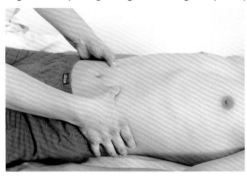

Fig.2-48　Opening four gates-
Huaroumen(ST24)

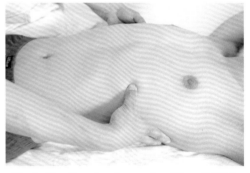

Fig.2-49　Opening four gates-*Riyue*(GB24)

manipulation on the points: *Shangwan*(CV13), *Zhongwan*(CV12), *Xiawan*(CV10) in line for 1 minute. Each point should be pushed and pointed for 5 to 10 seconds. (Fig.2-50)

(4) *Tonifying Shenque*(CV8)

Pressing the point *Shenque*(CV8) with the the thumbs overlapping, operate vibrating manipulation on it. The palm vibrating manipulation on point *Laogong*(PC8) pressing the point *Shenque*(CV8) is also used.(Fig.2-51)

(5) *Point penetrating Tianshu*(ST25)

Pointing the *Tianshu*(ST25) on both sides with both thumbs or middle fingers, put force

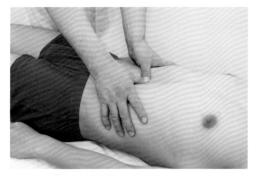

Fig.2-50 Pointing three wan

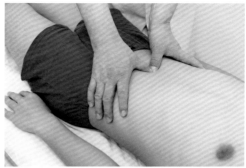

Fig.2-51 Tonifying *Shenque*(CV8)

to the contralateral side for 1 minute.(Fig.2-52)

(6) *Promoting Qihai*(CV6)

Performing the pointing manipulation and pushing manipulation with middle fingertip on point *Qihai*(CV6) for 1 minute.(Fig.2-53)

(7) *Lifting and shaking the abdomen*

Lifting the middle line region of the abdomen, smooth out the area with fingers from top to bottom combined with the shaking manipulation for 5-10 times. (Fig.2-54)

(8) *Circular rubbing the abdomen gently*

Circular rubbing the abdomen gently for 49 times, clockwise. And if the patient has

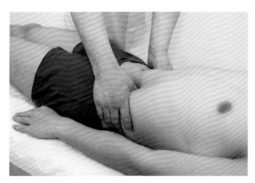

Fig.2-52 Point penetrating *Tianshu*(ST25)

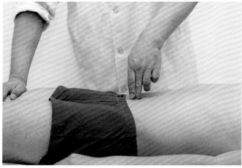

Fig.2-53 Promoting *Qihai*(CV6)

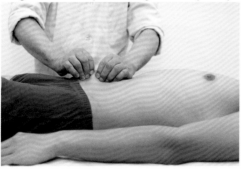

Fig.2-54 Lifting and shaking the abdomen

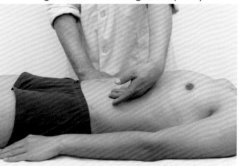

Fig.2-55 Circular rubbing the abdomen Ⅰ

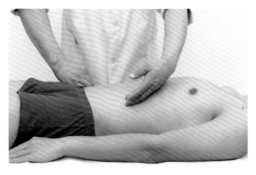

Fig.2-56 Circular rubbing the abdomen II

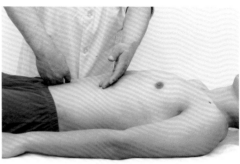

Fig.2-57 Circular rubbing the abdomen III

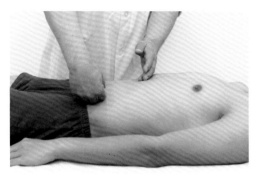

Fig.2-58 Circular rubbing the abdomen IV

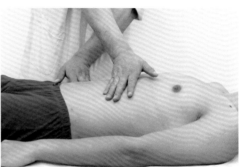

Fig.2-59 Circular rubbing the abdomen V

diarrhea, then circular rub the abdomen gently for 49 times, counterclockwise. (Fig.2-55 to Fig.2-59)

2.3.1.2 The pushing manipulation

We can see the pushing manipulation applied on the abdomen in Fig.2-60 to Fig.2-67.

2.3.1.3 The linear rubbing manipulation

We can see the linear rubbing manipulation applied on the abdomen in Fig.2-68, Fig.2-69.

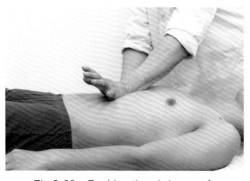

Fig.2-60 Pushing the abdomen I

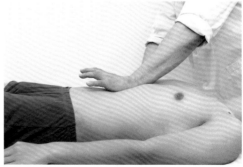

Fig.2-61 Pushing the abdomen II

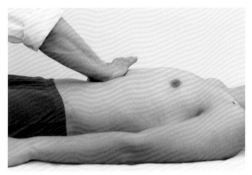
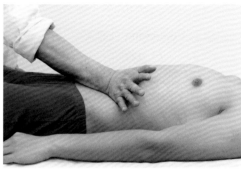

Fig.2-62　Backward pushing the abdomen Ⅰ　　Fig.2-63　Backward pushing the abdomen Ⅱ

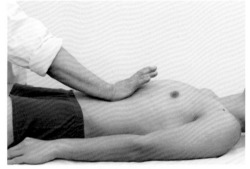
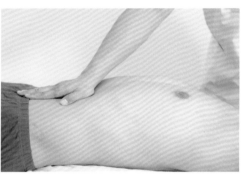

Fig.2-64　Backward pushing the abdomen Ⅲ　　Fig.2-65　Pushing conception vessel

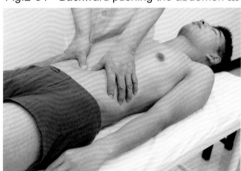
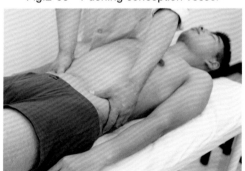

Fig.2-66　Separate pushing the abdomen Ⅰ　　Fig.2-67　Separate pushing the abdomen Ⅱ

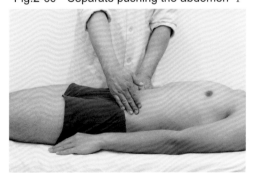
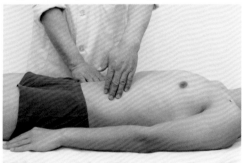

Fig.2-68　Linear rubbing the abdomen Ⅰ　　Fig.2-69　Linear rubbing the abdomen Ⅱ

2.3.1.4　The pointing manipulation

We can see the pointing manipulation applied on the sternum, *Tiantu*(CV22), *Tiwei*(EX-CA2) in Fig.2-70 to Fig.2-72.

2.3.1.5　Rubbing the flanks

We can see rubbing the flanks manipulation applied on the abdomen in Fig.2-73.

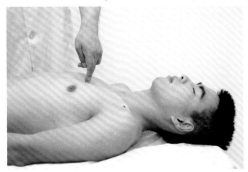

Fig.2-70　Pointing the sternum

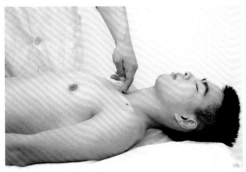

Fig.2-71　Pointing *Tiantu*(CV22)

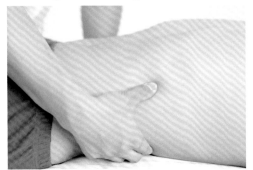

Fig.2-72　Pointing *Tiwei*(EX-CA2)(see in "Gastroptosis")

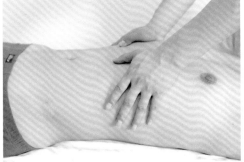

Fig.2-73　Rubbing the flanks

2.3.1.6　The kneading manipulation

We can see the kneading manipulation applied on the abdomen in Fig.2-74, Fig.2-75.

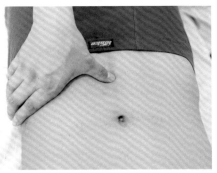

Fig.2-74　Kneading *Guanyuan*(GV4)

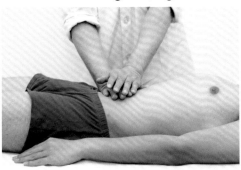

Fig.2-75　Kneading the abdomen

2.3.1.7 Concentrating the abdominal region

We can see the concentrating manipulation applied on the abdominal region in Fig.2-76, Fig.2-77.

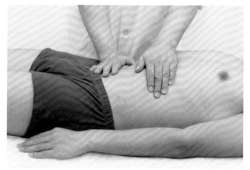

Fig.2-76 Concentrating the abdominal region Ⅰ

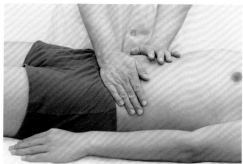

Fig.2-77 Concentrating the abdominal region Ⅱ

2.3.1.8 The pressing manipulation

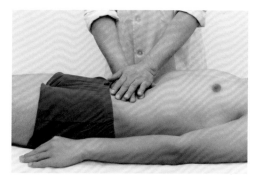

Fig.2-78 Pressing on the abdomen

We can see the pressing manipulation applied on the abdomen in Fig.2-78.

2.3.2 Cases of syndrome differentiation for clinical tuina manipulations

The following diseases should be treated based on the basic tuina manipulations applied on the thoracic and abdominal region first. And then according to the patterns of syndrome, add or subtract the following manipulations. (Note: Manipulations applied on the other part of the body will be narrated in other sections)

2.3.2.1 Gastroptosis

Perform the "Cui's eight tuina manipulations used on the abdomen" and the "Cui's six tuina manipulations used on the back" first.

And then, use the pointing and pressing method on the points *Tiwei*(EX-CA2), *Jiexi*(ST41), *Taichong*(LR3), *Sanyinjiao*(SP6), *Zusanli*(ST36), *Hegu*(LI4), *Neiguan*(PC6), *Quchi*(LI11). Pushing upward on the whole abdominal region with the thumb or root of the palm (this is also called backward pushing manipulation). Focus on pointing and pressing the point *Zusanli*(ST36) and *Neiguan*(PC6), kneading and pressing the points with thumb or middle finger for 20-30 times.

2.3.2.2 Constipation

Operate the "Cui's eight tuina manipulations used on the abdomen" first, and then adopt the following manipulations on the basis of syndrome differentiation.

Point the following points: *Zusanli*(ST36), *Sanyinjiao*(SP6), *Taichong*(LR3), *Zhigou*(TE 6), *Fenglong*(ST40), *Dachangshu*(BL25), *Pishu*(BL20), *Quchi*(LI11); Point the points: *Yunmen*(LU2), *Zhongfu*(LU1), *Danzhong*(CV17), *Zhangmen*(LR13), *Qimen*(LR14), *Feishu*(BL13), *Geshu*(BL17), *Ganshu*(BL18), etc. Lifting and shaking the abdomen, grasping and kneading the abdomen.

2.3.2.3 Diarrhea

Operate the "Cui's eight tuina manipulations used on the abdomen" first, and then adopt the following manipulations on the basis of syndrome differentiation.

Point the points *Qihai*(CV6), *Guanyuan*(CV4), *Zusanli*(ST36), circular rubbing the abdomen gently, counterclockwise; Point the points *Guanyuan*(CV4), *Qihai*(CV6), linear rubbing manipulation on the governor vessel, *Shenshu*(BL23), *Mingmen*(GV4), *Baliao*(BL31-BL34) and penetrate the warm into the region deeply by rubbing; Press and knead the points: *Zhangmen*(LR13), *Qimen*(LR14), *Ganshu*(BL18), *Danshu*(BL19), *Taichong*(LR3), *Xingjian*(LR2).

2.3.2.4 Dysmenorrhea

The important regions to treat dysmenorrhea are the points located on the abdomen, lumbar region and *Guanyuan*(CV4), *Qihai*(CV6), *Zhongji*(CV3), *Baliao*(BL31-BL34), *Zusanli*(ST36), *Sanyinjiao*(SP6). The manipulations operated on the abdomen should be gentle and soft. If there was serious spasm or pain in the abdomen, pointing and pressing points *Zusanli*(ST36) and *Sanyinjiao*(SP6) should be done first for about 1 minute to relieve the pain. And then perform the manipulations used on the abdomen. The manipulations used on the abdomen should be operated from outside to inside, the force should increase gradually, and the movement should be gentle and slow.

Commonly used manipulations

Linear rubbing on the lumbar and sacrum regions. Press and knead the points: *Shenshu* (BL23), *Ganshu*(BL18), *Geshu*(BL17), *Pishu*(BL20), *Weishu*(BL21), *Xuehai*(SP10), *Sanyinjiao*(SP6), *Ligou*(LR5), *Taichong*(LR3), *Baliao*(BL31-BL34). Scrap the costal arch. Separating yin and yang of the abdomen. Push points: *Zhongwan*(CV12), *Tianshu*(ST25), *Zusanli*(ST36).

2.3.2.5 Irregular menstruation

In the treatment of irregular menstruation, the "Cui's tuina manipulations used on the abdomen and back" is used mainly to regulate and tonify liver and kidney, tonify deficiency and dredge the channels.

Commonly used manipulations

Use circular rubbing the abdomen, clockwise. Circular kneading the abdomen, clockwise. Operating the "Whorl side thumb pushing manipulation" on the points: *Guanyuan*(CV4), *Qihai*(CV6). Press and knead the points: *Zusanli*(ST36), *Sanyinjiao*(SP6), *Ganshu*(BL18), *Pishu*(BL20), *Shenshu*(BL23), *Mingmen*(GV4), *Baliao*(BL31-BL34).

2.4　Tuina manipulations applied on the back and waist

2.4.1　Basic tuina manipulations applied on the back and waist

2.4.1.1　The "Cui's six tuina manipulations applied on the back"

(1) *Pointing manipulation along the five lines*

The five lines are the governor vessel line in the middle and the two branches of the bladder meridian of foot-*taiyang* on each side of the back. With the three fingers of the left hand pressing the middle finger of the right hand, the middle finger, index finger and ring finger of the right hand close to each other and operate the pointing manipulation on the intervertebral spaces for 3 to 5 times along the governor vessel line. And then, the middle finger and index finger of both hands perform the pointing manipulation on the branches of the bladder meridian of foot-*taiyang* on each side of the back together. (Fig.2-79; Fig.2-80)

(2) *Backward spine pinching*

Perform the spine pinching manipulation from the coccyx region to the point *Dazhui*(GV14) with the four fingers pressing forward and the thumb supporting the skin of both hands. Do not lift the skin in the first three whole line operation times. For the forth and fifth

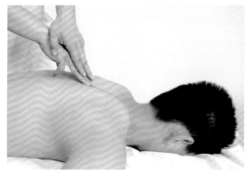
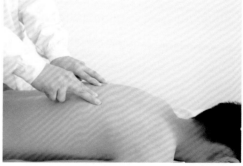

Fig.2-79　Pointing manipulation along the five lines Ⅰ

Fig.2-80　Pointing manipulation along the five lines Ⅱ

whole line operation, pinching three times and then lifting once until moving to the twelfth thoracic vertebra. The whole manipulation should be done for 5 times. (Fig.2-81)

(3) *Pushing manipulation on the three meridians*

Pushing and circular rubbing manipulation operated on the governor vessel and the bladder meridian of foot-*taiyang*.(Fig.2-82)

(4) *Pushing the region Baliao(BL31-BL34)*

With the point *Laogong*(PC8) in the palm press the region *Baliao*(BL31-BL34), while the manipulator focuses his/her mind on the point *Laogong*(PC8), steady the breathing and calm the nerves, touching the palate with the tip of tongue, push from the point *Changqiang*(GV1) to the region *Baliao*(BL31-BL34) for 300 to 500 times.(Fig.2-83)

(5) *Grasping the point Jianjing(GB21)*

Perform the grasping manipulation on the point *Jianjing*(GB21) for 3 to 5 times.(Fig.2-84)

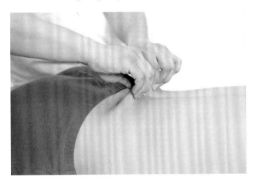

Fig.2-81　Backward spine pinching

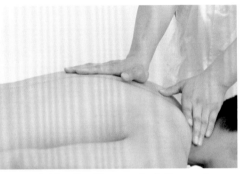

Fig.2-82　Pushing manipulation on the three meridians

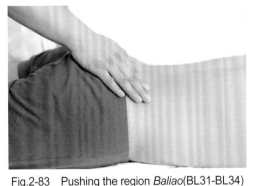

Fig.2-83　Pushing the region *Baliao*(BL31-BL34)

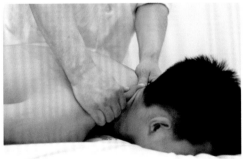

Fig.2-84　Grasping the point *Jianjing*(GB21)

(6) *Pushing the point Dazhui(GV14)*

Perform the pushing manipulation on the point *Dazhui*(GV14) for 3 to 5 times. It can be performed with the grasping manipulation on the point *Jianjing*(GB21) together.

2.4.1.2　Rolling manipulation

We can see the rolling manipulation applied on the back and waist in Fig.2-85 to Fig.2-92.

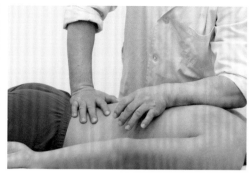

Fig.2-85   Erect rolling manipulation

Fig.2-86   Forearm rolling manipulation Ⅰ

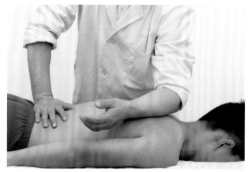

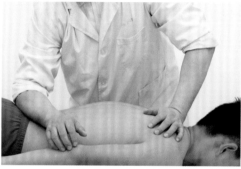

Fig.2-87   Forearm rolling manipulation Ⅱ

Fig.2-88   Forearm rolling manipulation Ⅲ

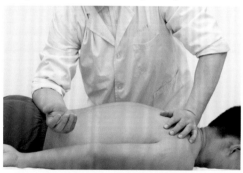

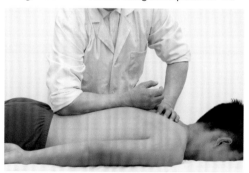

Fig.2-89   Forearm rolling manipulation Ⅳ

Fig.2-90   Forearm rolling manipulation Ⅴ

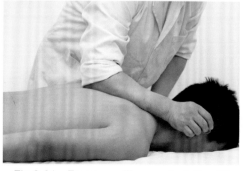

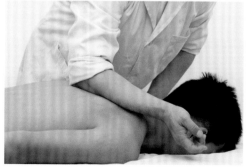

Fig.2-91   Forearm rolling manipulation Ⅵ

Fig.2-92   Forearm rolling manipulation Ⅶ

2.4.1.3 Flicking manipulation

We can see the flicking manipulation applied on the back in Fig.2-93.

2.4.1.4 Linear rubbing manipulation

We can see the linear rubbing manipulation applied on the back and waist in Fig.2-94 to Fig.2-96.

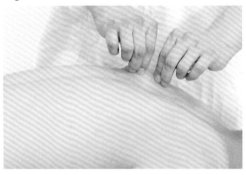

Fig.2-93   Flicking manipulation

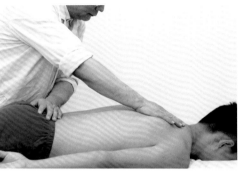

Fig.2-94   Linear rubbing manipulation Ⅰ

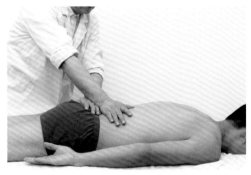

Fig.2-95   Linear rubbing manipulation Ⅱ

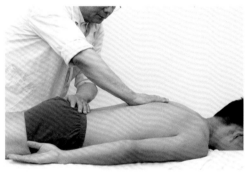

Fig.2-96   Linear rubbing manipulation Ⅲ

2.4.1.5 Plucking manipulation

We can see the plucking manipulation applied on the back and waist in Fig.2-97, Fig.2-98.

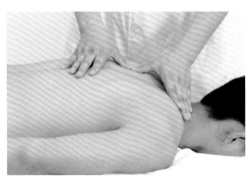

Fig.2-97   Plucking manipulation with thumbs

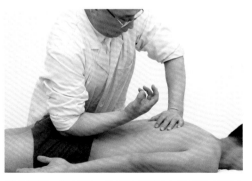

Fig.2-98   Plucking manipulation with the elbow

2.4.1.6　Pressing manipulation

We can see the pressing manipulation applied on the back and waist in Fig.2-99, Fig.2-100.

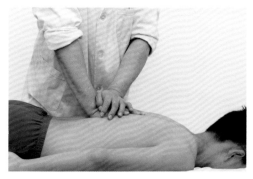
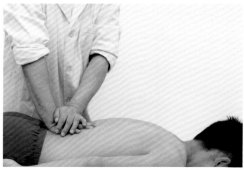

Fig.2-99　Pressing manipulation Ⅰ　　　　　Fig.2-100　Pressing manipulation Ⅱ

2.4.1.7　Patting manipulation

We can see the patting manipulation applied on the back and waist in Fig.2-101, Fig.2-102.

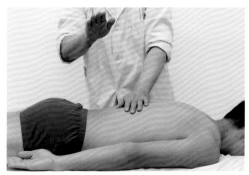
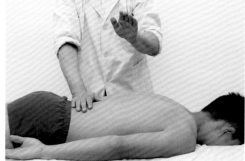

Fig.2-101　Patting the back　　　　　　Fig.2-102　Patting the waist

2.4.1.8　Tapping manipulation

We can see the tapping manipulation applied on the back and waist in Fig.2-103, Fig.2-104.

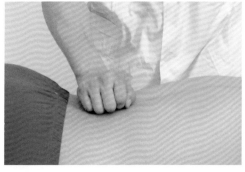
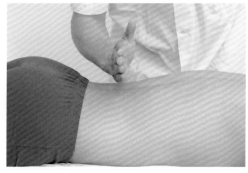

Fig.2-103　Tapping manipulation with a soft fist　　Fig.2-104　Side hitting manipulation

2.4.1.9　Kneading manipulation

We can see the kneading manipulation applied on the back and waist in Fig.2-105, Fig.2-106.

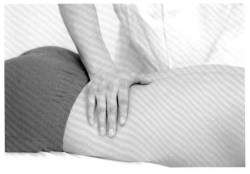
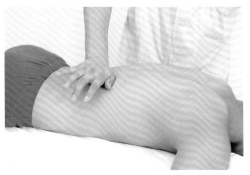

Fig.2-105　Palm kneading manipulation　　　Fig.2-106　Heel of hand kneading manipulation

2.4.1.10　Pinching manipulation

We can see the pinching manipulation applied on the back and waist in Fig.2-107 to Fig.2-109.

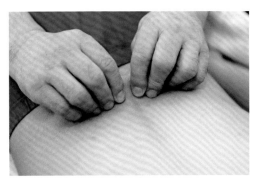
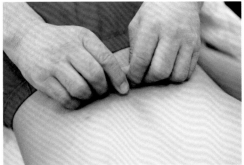

Fig.2-107　Three-fingers pinching manipulation Ⅰ　　　Fig.2-108　Three-fingers pinching manipulation Ⅱ

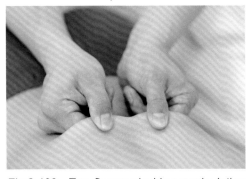

Fig.2-109　Two-fingers pinching manipulation

2.4.1.11　Pointing manipulation

We can see the pointing the point *Xinshu*(BL15) on the back and *Mingmen*(GV4) on the waist in Fig.2-110, Fig.2-111.

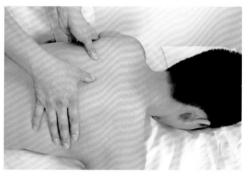 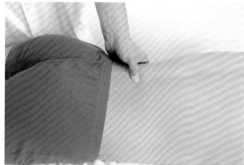

Fig.2-110　Pointing the point *Xinshu*(BL15)　　Fig.2-111　Pointing the point *Mingmen*(GV4)

2.4.2　Other tuina manipulations applied on the back and waist

2.4.2.1　Cross pressing reduction manipulation on the back with the palm

The patient takes the prone position. The doctor, with crossed arms, places the heels of the hands on both sides of the spinal process and tells the patient to take a deep breath, apply a sudden outward and downward force at the end of the exhale, a successful reduction is marked with a cracking sound. (Fig.2-112)

Operational requirements

The sudden force applied by the hands should be appropriate and the hand on the tilted side of the spine closer inward the other and apply less force than the other.

The main applicable regions

Joints of thoracic vertebrae.

Cautions

The sudden force applied should be appropriate, and the heels of hands fixed to the patient's back, the therapist should keep the body steady and breath even, and the snapping sound is not always necessary.

2.4.2.2　Pressing and pushing manipulation on the patient in prone position

The patient takes prone position, naturally relaxed, and the therapist stands at the patient side and puts his right hand on the affected spinous process, then with the left hand on the back of the right hand, the therapist then tells the patient to take a deep breath, and at the end of the exhale, make a small scale downward pushing movement and the sound of joint reduction should be heard. Suitable for reduction of middle and lower spine joints. (Fig.2-113)

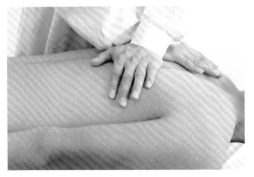

Fig.2-112　Cross pressing reduction manipulation on the back with the palm

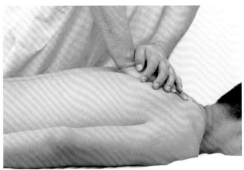

Fig.2-113　Pressing and pushing manipulation on the patient in prone position

2.4.2.3　The thoracic vertebrae reduction manipulation in supine position

The doctor should tell the patient to stand and stoop, and then feel the thoracic vertebrae for the tilted spot, after that the doctor should tell the patient to take supine position in bed with arms crossed in front of the chest. With one hand forming a halfway fist and placed on both sides of the tilted spinal process and the other hand securing the patient's crossed arms, the doctor should tell the patient to breath and relax while slightly press against the patient's chest, when the patient is thoroughly relaxed, apply a sudden force. A successful reduction is marked with a cracking sound. (Fig.2-114 to Fig.2-116) Also fit to press a knee against the tilted spinal process for reduction. (Fig.2-117)

Operational requirements

Locating should be precise, press steadily, accurately, and deftly, apply force at the maximum limit.

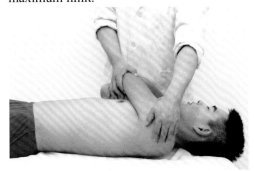

Fig.2-114　The thoracic vertebrae reduction manipulation in supine position Ⅰ

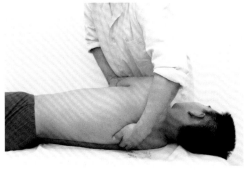

Fig.2-115　The thoracic vertebrae reduction manipulation in supine position Ⅱ

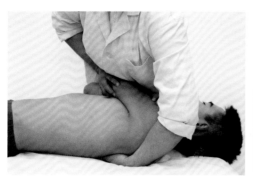 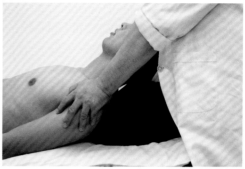

Fig.2-116　The thoracic vertebrae reduction manipulation in supine position III

Fig.2-117　The thoracic vertebrae reduction manipulation in supine position IV

Cautions

When applying the treatment, if not successful at one try, do not repeat the treatment, apply some tendon regulating, grasping, point pressing, rubbing, kneading or other spasm relieving manipulations, and then perform the reduction manipulation. Some patients may need 4 to 5 rounds of treatment, applied once in a few days, do not rush it. In the application of this treatment, locating is the key, the reduction should be precise, the force should be soft, never violent. Do not blindly push for the cracking sound.

2.4.2.4　The lifting thoracic vertebrae reduction manipulation with chest out

The patient takes a standing position, fingers clasped together docked at the neck. The doctor should stand behind the patient, hands through the patient's underarm and passing through the chelidon and grasping the patient's forearms. Then tell the patient to relax and lean against the doctor's chest, with hands and waist working together, apply a sudden lifting force and lift the chest to make reduction. Suitable for reduction of upper thoracic spine. (Fig.2-118)

2.4.2.5　The knee thoracic vertebrae reduction manipulation in sitting position

The patient should be sitting on a square stool, fingers clasped together and docked at the neck against. The doctor should be behind the patient, holding the patient's elbows with both hands, and knee against the tilted spinal process, pull slowly backwards to the maximum limit, and apply a sudden force, a cracking sound should be heard. Suitable for middle and upper thoracic spine. (Fig.2-119)

2.4.2.6　Oblique wrenching manipulation of the lumbar vertebrae

The patient takes a lateral position on the unaffected side, head tilts back and lays even on a pillow, leg on the unaffected side straightened and stretched with the other leg flexed on top (adjust the flexed leg's position according to the subluxation position), arm on the unaffected side straightened and stretched in front of the chest and the other arm flexed behind; the doctor should stand at the patient's abdomen side with one hand (or upper arm) on the front side of the affected side shoulder, and the other arm flexed (or use hand) on the back side of the hip of the affected side. The doctor should apply and gradually build up opposite forces to rotate the affected area to the maximum limit and before applying a sudden force (pushing mainly on the hip, not the shoulder) and exceed the rotate limit. A successful reduction is marked with a cracking sound. (Fig.2-120; Fig.2-121)

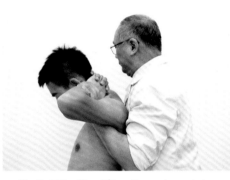

Fig.2-118　The lifting thoracic vertebrae reduction manipulation with chest out

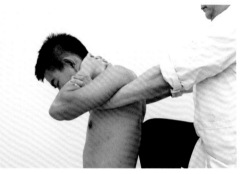

Fig.2-119　The knee thoracic vertebrae reduction manipulation in sitting position

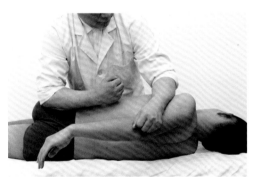

Fig.2-120　Oblique wrenching manipulation of the lumbar vertebrae Ⅰ

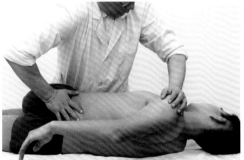

Fig.2-121　Oblique wrenching manipulation of the lumbar vertebrae Ⅱ

Operational requirements

Locating should be precise, press steadily, accurate, and deftly, apply force at the maximum limit.

Cautions

When applying the treatment, if not successful at one try, do not repeat the treatment, do not pursue quick results. locate the affected spin precisely, and the reduction should be precise and soft, do not rush for the cracking sound.

2.4.2.7 Wrenching leg and pressing waist manipulation

The doctor should press against the patient's waist with one hand and hold the contralateral thigh 1/3 lower with the other hand and wrench the leg upward and backward. With two hands working together, one pushing downward against the waist and the other lift the leg upward, shake the leg before lower it slowly; repeat the same procedures 3 to 5 times and move to the other side. (Fig.2-122)

2.4.2.8 Wrenching shoulder and pressing waist manipulation

The doctor should push against the patient's waist with one hand and hold the front side of the contralateral shoulder with the other hand. With two hands working together, one pushing downward against the waist and the other hand wrenching the shoulder upward, when the waist is flexed to the maximum limit and relaxed, apply a sudden force and then lower it slowly. (Fig.2-123)

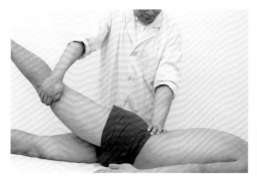 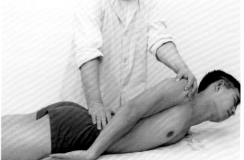

Fig.2-122　Wrenching leg and pressing waist manipulation   Fig.2-123　Wrenching shoulder and pressing waist manipulation

2.4.2.9 Three times tapping manipulation (applied to treat "acute lumbar sprain")

The patient takes prone position, hands push against the treatment couch, try every possible effort to do push-ups, and the doctor should support the patient by the right hand holding the abdomen upward. When the patient lift to the maximum limit, the doctor should strike the patient's lumbar with a firm force by the left half palm and at the same time withdrawing force (not the hand) from the left hand causing the patient to lie onto the bed, repeat 3 times. (Fig.2-124 to Fig.2-126)

2.4.2.10 Bending hip and knee manipulation (applied to treat "acute lumbar sprain")

Tell the patient to turn over and lie flat while bending both the hip and knee, the doctor should hold the ankles with one hand and knees with the other, bend the knees close to

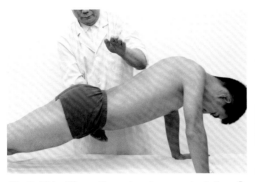

Fig.2-124　Three times tapping manipulation Ⅰ

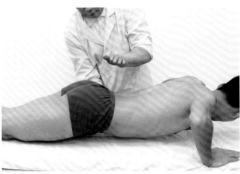

Fig.2-125　Three times tapping manipulation Ⅱ

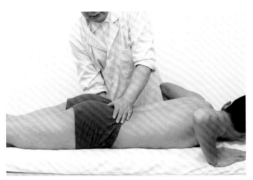

Fig.2-126　Three times tapping manipulation Ⅲ

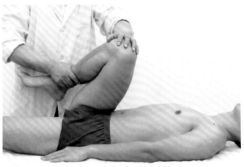

Fig.2-127　Bending hip and knee
manipulation Ⅰ

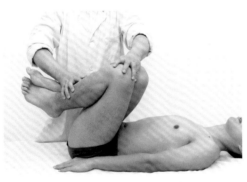

Fig.2-128　Bending hip and knee
manipulation Ⅱ

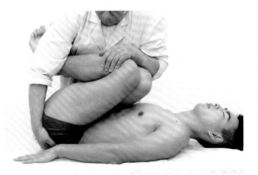

Fig.2-129　Bending hip and knee
manipulation Ⅲ

the chest and do some left and right rotating first, gradually increasing the movement scale, and then push the knees forward and downward so the waist would be over bent and lifted from the bed, repeat for several times. (Fig.2-127 to Fig.2-129)

2.4.2.11　Pulling and shaking the waist manipulation

The patient takes prone position, and the doctor should stand by the patient's feet, hold the patient's ankles with both hands, pull in the direction of the vertical axis first till the

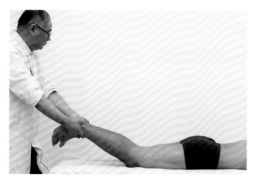
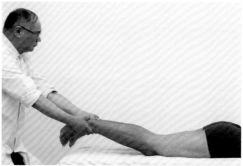

Fig.2-130　Pulling and shaking the waist manipulation Ⅰ

Fig.2-131　Pulling and shaking the waist manipulation Ⅱ

patient is relaxed, pull upward and shake with a sudden force, send a wave down the patient's body so the patient's waist is lifted off the bed, repeat for 3 times. (Fig.2-130; Fig.2-131)

2.4.2.12　The hip and knee bending reduction manipulation (applied to treat "sacroiliac joint dysfunction")

Tell the patient to take the supine position and relax with lower limbs stretched out with a pillow under the waist. The doctor should stand at the patient's affected side, hold the ankle with one hand and secure the knee of the affected limb with the other, gradually bend the hip and knee to the maximum limit and tell the patient to inhale deeply and then exhale, at the end of the exhale, apply a sudden downward force and over bend the hip joint, a joint reduction sound should be heard if successful. If so, tell the patient to stretch the affected limb. (Fig.2-132 to Fig.2-137)

2.4.2.13　Extending stretching reduction manipulation (applied to treat "sacroiliac joint dysfunction")

When performing, the doctor takes a lunge standing position. With one hand holding the

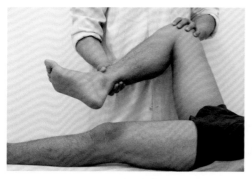
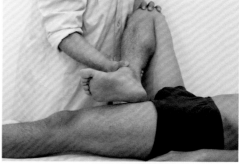

Fig.2-132　The hip and knee bending reduction manipulation Ⅰ

Fig.2-133　The hip and knee bending reduction manipulation Ⅱ

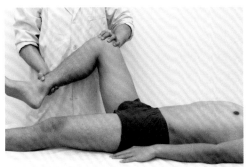

Fig.2-134　The hip and knee bending reduction manipulation III

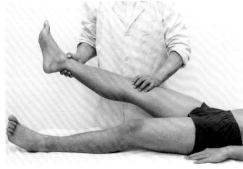

Fig.2-135　The hip and knee bending reduction manipulation IV

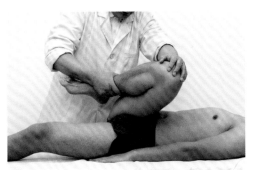

Fig.2-136　The hip and knee bending reduction manipulation V

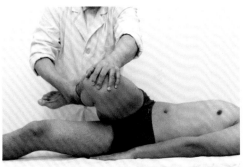

Fig.2-137　The hip and knee bending reduction manipulation VI

knee of the affected side and the other hand grasping the ankle of the same leg, bend the hip joint and knee to the maximum limit. Tell the patient to be relaxed and breathe naturally. The patient extends the affected limb gradually to coordinate the doctor's movement. And then, the doctor stretches the flexing affected limb to straight and suddenly with the force, so as to drive the homolateral ilium by the manipulation. (Fig.2-138)

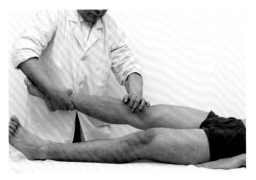

Fig.2-138　Extending stretching reduction manipulation

2.4.2.14　Pulling and pressing manipulation on the patient in prone position (applied to treat "sacroiliac joint dysfunction")

The patient takes a prone position on the bed with a thin cushion under abdomen and grasping the bedside. An assistant stands at the end of the bed with hands grasping the patient's ankle of the affected side. Then, pulls the leg, and hold the traction. The operator puts the root part of the hand on the bulge part of the sacroiliac joint on the affected side, tells the patient to breathe deeply. And at the end of patient's expiration, the operator presses downward and outward suddenly to make the ilium reduction following the direction of the force generated by the operator. Cracking sounds or subjectivity of sacroiliac movement show the success reduction of the manipulation. (Fig.2-139)

2.4.2.15 Pushing and pressing manipulation on the patient with the hip joint in hyperextension in side-lying position (applied to treat "sacroiliac joint dysfunction")

Patient Lies on the side with the affected side upwards. And the operator stands by the back of the patient. With the bottom of hand against the bulge part of the sacroiliac joint on the affected side, push it forward. Meanwhile, the knee on the affected side is required to be bent. And the operator grasps the patient's the ankle of the affected side, stretching backwards for the hip joint in hyperextension on the affected side. Push and pull several times with both hands, wait the patient relaxed, push and press with increasing force to make the hip joint in hyperextension for one time, so as to make the ilium on the affected side rotate forward into reduction. (Fig.2-140)

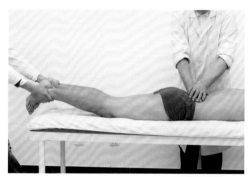 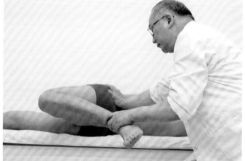

Fig.2-139 Pulling and pressing manipulation on the patient in prone position

Fig.2-140 Pushing and pressing manipulation on the patient with the hip joint in hyperextension in side-lying position

2.4.2.16 Shaking waist manipulation on the patient in sitting position

The patient takes the sitting position. The doctor stands behind the patient and then tells the patient to lean back with the doctor's hand holding the patient's shoulder. With an assistant fixing the patient's knee, the patient leaning back to a certain angle until the affected lumbar vertebrae moving, the doctor shakes the patient's lumbar by the force from the lumbar muscles. (Fig.2-141 to Fig.2-143)

2.4.2.17 Wrenching manipulation for locating and rotating lumbar vertebrae

The patient takes the sitting position. The doctor stands in front of the patient and near the affected side, holds the patient's huckle by both legs. Put hands on patient's shoulders each, wrenching the patient to make the lumbar vertebrae rotating to the affected side. When the patient's lumbar vertebrae turns to a certain angle until the affected vertebrae is moving, rotate it with a sudden increase force, and then relax. The cracking sound will be heard to show the reduction manipulation to the facet joint of the lumbar vertebrae is success. (Fig.2-144 to Fig.2-146)

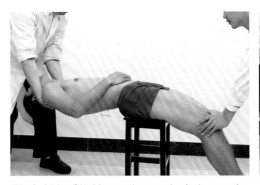

Fig.2-141　Shaking waist manipulation on the patient in sitting position Ⅰ

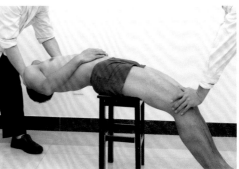

Fig.2-142　Shaking waist manipulation on the patient in sitting position Ⅱ

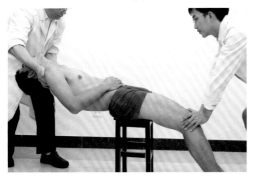

Fig.2-143　Shaking waist manipulation on the patient in sitting position Ⅲ

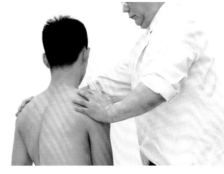

Fig.2-144　Wrenching manipulation for locating and rotating lumbar vertebrae Ⅰ

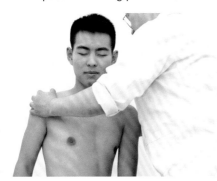

Fig.2-145　Wrenching manipulation for locating and rotating lumbar vertebrae Ⅱ

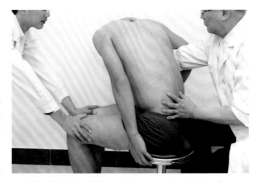

Fig.2-146　Wrenching manipulation for locating and rotating lumbar vertebrae Ⅲ

2.4.2.18 Back-carrying manipulation

The back-carrying manipulation means the operator carrying the patient, back to back or back to side in order to pull and vibrate the lumbar vertebrae. The operator carries the patient with the force against the patient's waist. As a traditional tuina therapy, it has an obvious effect on lumbar diseases like acute lumbar sprain, etc. (Fig.2-147; Fig.2-148)

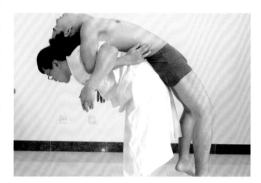
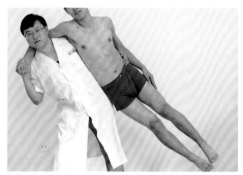

Fig.2-147　Back-carrying manipulation Ⅰ　　　Fig.2-148　Back-carrying manipulation Ⅱ

2.4.3　Cases of syndrome differentiation for clinical tuina manipulations

According to clinical syndromes, there are some routine treatment manipulations for lumbodorsal disorders, and they are consisted by the above-mentioned manipulations. The following manipulations are for reference. (Note: Manipulations applied on the other part of the body will be narrated in other sections)

2.4.3.1 Back myofascitis

Commonly used manipulations

Kneading and pressing manipulations. Rolling manipulations. Plucking manipulations. Pointing manipulations on the following points: *Huantiao*(GB30), *Weizhong*(BL40), *Chengshan*(BL57), *Shenshu*(BL23), ashi point (the painful point) on the lumbar region, *Fengchi*(GB20), *Tianzong*(SI11). Plucking the points: *Yanglingquan*(GB34). Patting manipulation.

2.4.3.2 Chronic lumbar muscle strain

Commonly used manipulations

Kneading and pressing manipulations. Rolling manipulations. Plucking manipulations. Pointing manipulations on the following points: *Huantiao*(GB30), *Weizhong*(BL40),

Chengshan(BL57), *Shenshu*(BL23), ashi point (the painful point) on the lumbar region. Pushing manipulation. Sweeping manipulation. Patting manipulation.

2.4.3.3 Lumbar spinal stenosis

Commonly used manipulations

Kneading manipulations. Rolling manipulations. Plucking manipulations. Pointing manipulations on the following points: *Huantiao*(GB30), *Weizhong*(BL40), *Yanglingquan* (GB34), *Kunlun*(BL60), *Taixi*(KI3). The rolling waist exercise with holding knees.

2.4.3.4 Lumbar spondylolisthesis

Commonly used manipulations

Palm kneading manipulations. Rolling manipulations. Plucking manipulations. Pointing manipulations on the following points: *Huantiao*(GB30), *Weizhong*(BL40), *Yanglingquan*(GB34), *Chengshan*(BL57), *Taixi*(KI3), *Kunlun*(BL60), *Shenque*(CV8), *Tianshu*(ST25). Palm pushing manipulation. Wrenching manipulation for locating and rotating lumbar vertebrae.

2.4.3.5 Acute lumbar sprain

Commonly used manipulations

Kneading manipulations. Rolling manipulations. Plucking manipulations. Pointing manipulations on the following points: *Yinmen*(BL37), *Weizhong*(BL40), *Yanglingquan* (GB34). Pointing toward to each other on *Taixi*(KI3) and *Kunlun*(BL 60).

Reduction techniques

In the treatment of acute lumbar sprain, especially for the treatment of acute lumbar posterior articular disturbance, the "Cui's 3+3+3 combined manipulations" have obvious effect and great feature. The first 3 is the "Three times tapping manipulation". The second 3 is three times wrenching manipulations include the "oblique wrenching manipulation of the lumbar vertebrae" on the left side and right side, the "bending hip and knee manipulation". The third 3 is pointing three times on three points include one point *Shenque*(CV8) in the governor vessel and two points *Tianshu*(ST25) in the bladder meridian of foot-*yangming* in each side.

2.4.3.6 Lumbar intervertebral disc protrusion

Commonly used manipulations

Plucking manipulations. Kneading manipulations. Rolling manipulations. Pushing manipulation. Pulling and shaking manipulation. Pointing manipulations on the following points: *Chengfu*(BL36), *Yinmen*(BL37), *Weizhong*(BL40), *Yanglingquan*(GB34), *Chengshan*(BL57), *Taixi*(KI3), Kunlun(BL60). The oblique wrenching manipulation of the lumbar vertebrae.

2.4.3.7 Sacroiliac joint dysfunction

Commonly used manipulations

Plucking manipulations. Kneading manipulations.

Reduction techniques

The hip and knee bending reduction manipulation. Extending stretching reduction manipulation. Pulling and pressing manipulation on the patient in prone position. Pushing and pressing manipulation on the patient with the hip joint in hyperextension in side-lying position.

2.5 Tuina manipulations applied on the shoulder

2.5.1 Basic tuina manipulations applied on the shoulder

2.5.1.1 Kneading manipulation

We can see the kneading manipulation applied on the shoulder in Fig.2-149 to Fig.2-151.

2.5.1.2 Pointing manipulation

We can see the pointing manipulation applied on the shoulder in Fig.2-152, Fig.2-153.

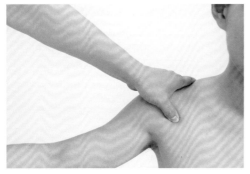 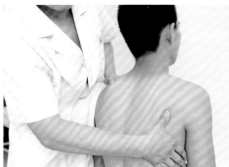

Fig.2-149 Kneading the interior of the shoulder   Fig.2-150 Kneading the outside of scapula

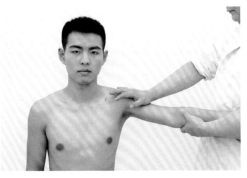

Fig.2-151   Kneading the shoulder with the heel of palm

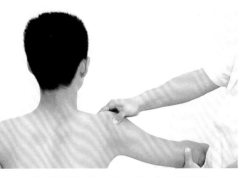

Fig.2-152   Pointing *Jianliao*(TE14)

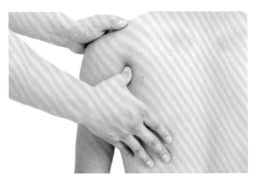

Fig.2-153   Pointing *Tianzong*(SI11)

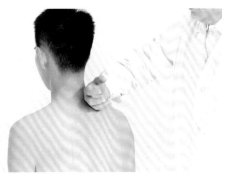

Fig.2-154   Side rolling manipulation on the shoulder Ⅰ

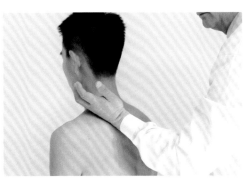

Fig.2-155   Side rolling manipulation on the shoulder Ⅱ

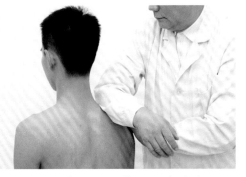

Fig.2-156   Forearm rolling manipulation on the shoulder Ⅰ

2.5.1.3   Rolling manipulation

We can see the rolling manipulation applied on the shoulder in Fig.2-154 to Fig.2-160.

2.5.1.4   Rotating manipulation

We can see the rotating manipulation applied on the shoulder in Fig.2-161 to Fig.2-168.

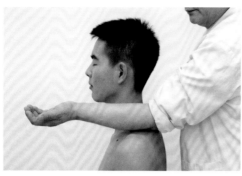

Fig.2-157　Forearm rolling manipulation on
the shoulder II

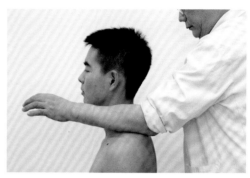

Fig.2-158　Forearm rolling manipulation on
the shoulder III

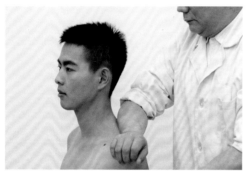

Fig.2-159　Forearm rolling manipulation on
the shoulder IV

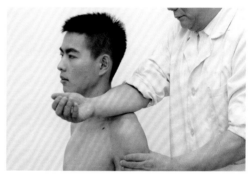

Fig.2-160　Forearm rolling manipulation on
the shoulder V

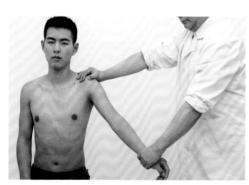

Fig.2-161　Rotating manipulation on the
shoulder I

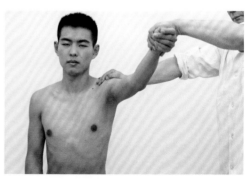

Fig.2-162　Rotating manipulation on the
shoulder II

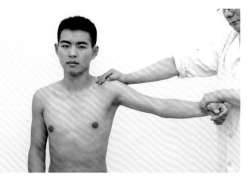

Fig.2-163   Rotating manipulation on the
shoulder III

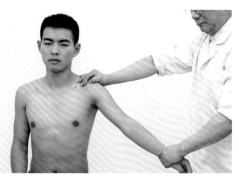

Fig.2-164   Rotating manipulation on the
shoulder IV

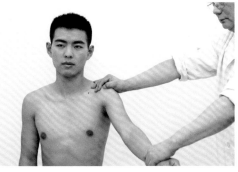

Fig.2-165   Rotating manipulation on the
shoulder V

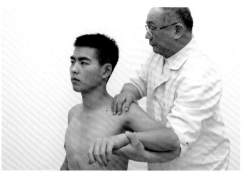

Fig.2-166   Rotating manipulation on the
shoulder VI

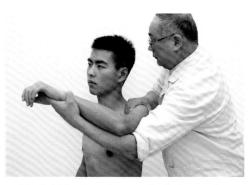

Fig.2-167   Rotating manipulation on the
shoulder VII

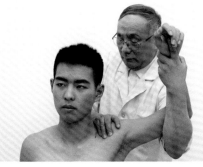

Fig.2-168   Rotating manipulation on the
shoulder VIII

2.5.1.5　Pulling-extending manipulation

We can see the pulling-extending manipulation applied on the shoulder in Fig.2-169 to Fig.2-172.

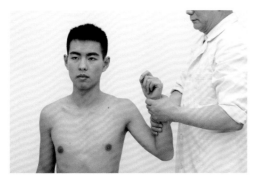

Fig.2-169　Pulling-extending manipulation on the shoulder Ⅰ

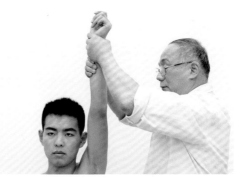

Fig.2-170　Pulling-extending manipulation on the shoulder Ⅱ

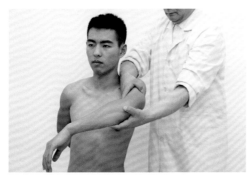

Fig.2-171　Pulling-extending manipulation on the shoulder Ⅲ

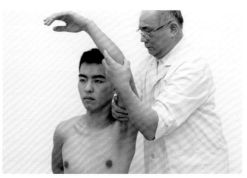

Fig.2-172　Pulling-extending manipulation on the shoulder Ⅳ

2.5.1.6　Moving manipulation

We can see the moving manipulation applied on the shoulder in Fig.2-173 to Fig.2-177.

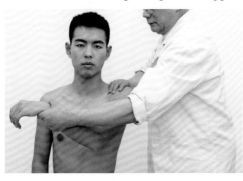

Fig.2-173　Adduction

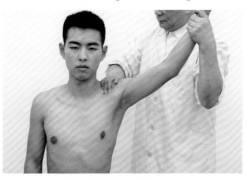

Fig.2-174　Abduction

2.5.1.7 Patting manipulation

We can see the patting manipulation applied on the shoulder in Fig.2-178 to Fig.2-181.

2.5.1.8 Knocking manipulation

We can see the knocking manipulation applied on the shoulder in Fig.2-182 to Fig.2-187.

2.5.1.9 Concentrating manipulation

We can see concentrating the shoulder manipulation in Fig.2-188.

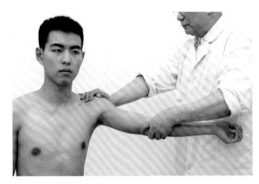

Fig.2-175　External rotating

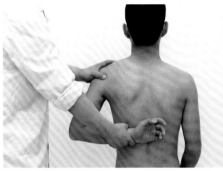

Fig.2-176　Posterior extension

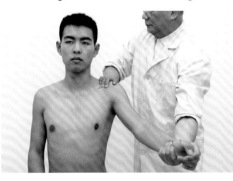

Fig.2-177　Anteflexion

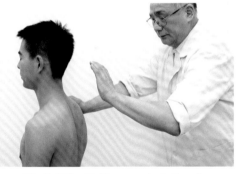

Fig.2-178　Patting manipulation Ⅰ

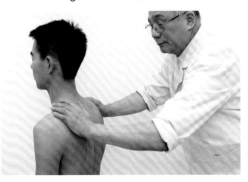

Fig.2-179　Patting manipulation Ⅱ

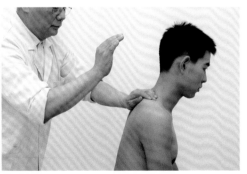

Fig.2-180　Patting manipulation Ⅲ

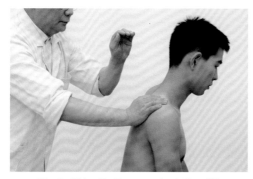

Fig.2-181　Patting manipulation IV

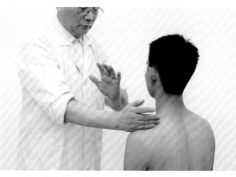

Fig.2-182　Knocking manipulation I

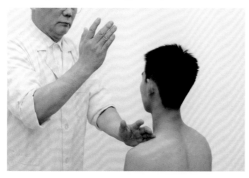

Fig.2-183　Knocking manipulation II

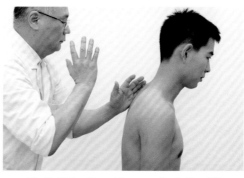

Fig.2-184　Knocking manipulation III

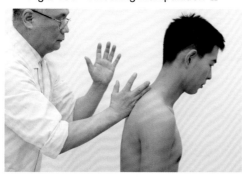

Fig.2-185　Knocking manipulation IV

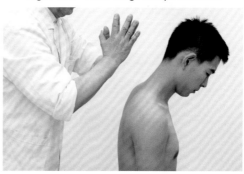

Fig.2-186　Knocking manipulation V

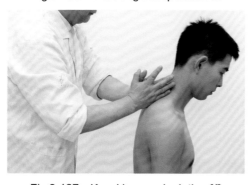

Fig.2-187　Knocking manipulation VI

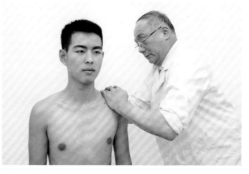

Fig.2-188　Concentrating the shoulder manipulation

2.5.1.10   Twisting manipulation

We can see twisting the shoulder manipulation in Fig.2-189.

2.5.1.11   Plucking manipulation

We can see the plucking manipulation applied on the shoulder in Fig.2-190.

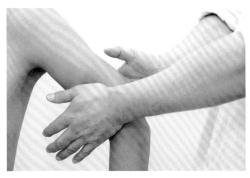

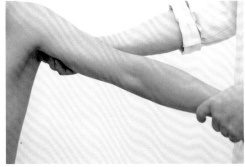

Fig.2-189   Twisting the shoulder manipulation   Fig.2-190   Plucking manipulation

2.5.1.12   Shaking manipulation

We can see the shaking manipulation applied on the shoulder in Fig.2-191.

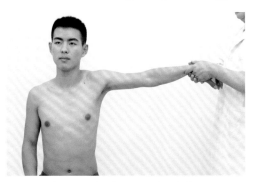

Fig.2-191   Shaking manipulation on
             the shoulder

2.5.2   Other tuina manipulations applied on the shoulder

2.5.2.1   The joint reduction manipulation in the treatment of shoulder joint subluxation

The patient is in the supine position. The operator sits beside the patient's affected side, holds the wrist of the affected limb. With the foot pushing patient's armpit of the affected limb, keep pulling the affected limb for 2 minutes. And then, an assistant takes the affected limb in the pulling condition, abducing and external rotating the upper arm to touch his/her ear and then adducting and internal rotating back to return the affected limb to the operator. The operator increases the angle of adduction and internal rotation, and a cracking sound will be heard to show the reduction is success. After the reduction, the forearm should be kept in a brace. The brace should surround the affected shoulder from underneath to the upper lateral side of shoulder. There should be a book or board under the affected forearm to fix the arm and uniformly forced. Adjust the length of the brace to keep the elbow flexed at 90°. Fix the arm for 3 days and avoid the affected arm exertion. (Fig.2-192 to Fig.2-196)

2.5.2.2　Passive pulling the shoulder joint

We can see the passive pulling the shoulder joint manipulation in Fig.2-197 to Fig.2-201.

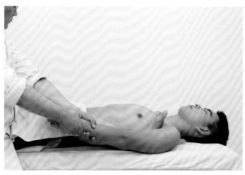
Fig.2-192　Shoulder joint subluxation Ⅰ

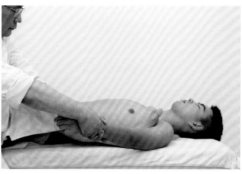
Fig.2-193　Shoulder joint subluxation Ⅱ

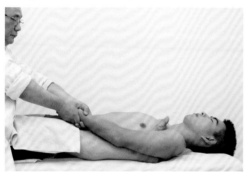
Fig.2-194　Shoulder joint subluxation Ⅲ

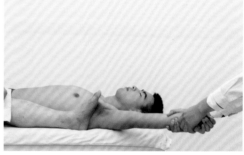
Fig.2-195　Shoulder joint subluxation Ⅳ

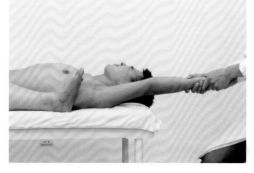
Fig.2-196　Shoulder joint subluxation Ⅴ

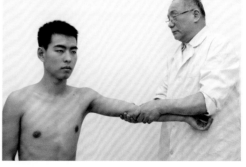
Fig.2-197　Passive pulling the shoulder joint Ⅰ

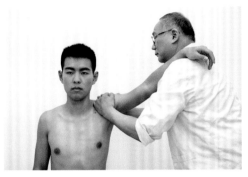

Fig.2-198 Passive pulling the shoulder joint Ⅱ

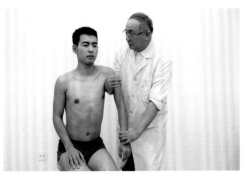

Fig.2-199 Passive pulling the shoulder joint Ⅲ

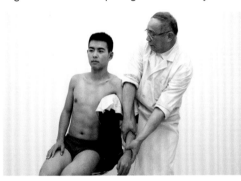

Fig.2-200 Passive pulling the shoulder joint Ⅳ

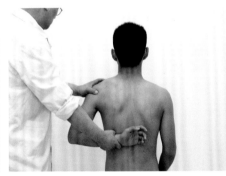

Fig.2-201 Passive pulling the shoulder joint Ⅴ

2.6 Tuina manipulations applied on the elbow

2.6.1 Basic tuina manipulations applied on the elbow

2.6.1.1 Kneading manipulation

We can see the kneading manipulation applied on the elbow in Fig.2-202, Fig.2-203.

2.6.1.2 Plucking manipulation

We can see the kneading manipulation applied on the elbow in Fig.2-204, Fig.2-205.

2.6.1.3 Moving manipulation

We can see the moving manipulation applied on the elbow in Fig.2-206 to Fig.2-208.

2.6.1.4 Pointing manipulation

We can see the pointing manipulation applied on the points *Shousanli*(LI10), *Quchi*(LI11) on the elbow in Fig.2-209, Fig.2-210.

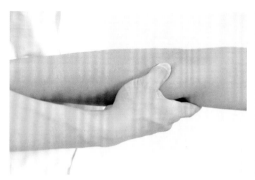

Fig.2-202　Thumb kneading manipulation

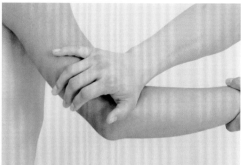

Fig.2-203　Palm kneading manipulation

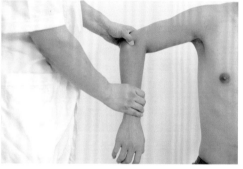

Fig.2-204　Plucking the radial side of elbow

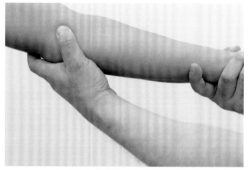

Fig.2-205　Plucking the ulnar side of elbow

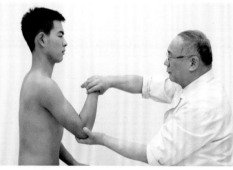

Fig.2-206　Flexing the elbow

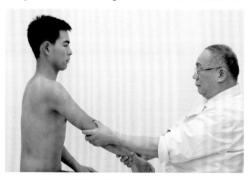

Fig.2-207　Extending the elbow

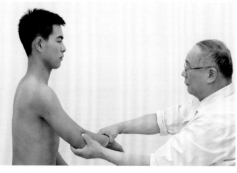

Fig.2-208　Adduction

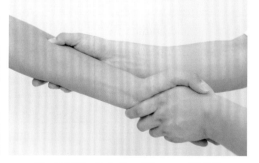

Fig.2-209　Pointing *Shousanli*(LI10)

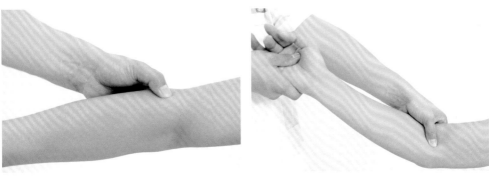

| Fig.2-210   Pointing *Quchi*(LI11) | Fig.2-211   Pressing the brachial artery |

2.6.1.5   Pressing manipulation

We can see the pressing manipulation applied on the elbow in Fig.2-211.

2.6.2   Cases of syndrome differentiation for clinical tuina manipulations

According to the clinical manifestation of the disease, the basic tuina manipulation should be flexible used. All the diseases can be treated based on an overall analysis of the illness and the patient's condition as the routine of the relaxing manipulations, the therapeutic manipulation and the finishing manipulation. (Note: Manipulations applied to other parts of the body will be narrated in other sections)

2.6.2.1   Lateral humeral epicondylitis

Pointing and pressing manipulation on the ashi point (the pain point), *Quchi*(LI11), *Jianjing*(GB21), *Shousanli*(LI10), *Hegu*(LI4). Each point should be pointed and pressed for half a minute.

(1) *Kneading manipulation*

The doctor should sit beside the patient's affected side, holding the affected arm with one hand. Circle knead the patient's affected arm from the outer side of the forearm, passing the elbow to the shoulder part gently and softly with the palm and fingers of the other hand. Perform the manipulation for 5 minutes. And then, the doctor changes the hand, with one hand holding the affected arm, and the other hand kneading from the inner side of the forearm passing the elbow to the armpit. Perform the manipulation for another 5 minutes. And focus on kneading and pointing the muscles around the elbow joint.

(2) *Plucking manipulation*

The doctor, with one hand holding the patient's wrist and making the palm upward, the other hand holding the patient's elbow with the thumb on the outer side of the elbow and the four fingers on the inner side, makes the patient's elbow joint doing the flexion and extension movement. Simultaneously, make an up and down vertical plucking manipulation on the lateral epicondyle of Humerus of the affected limb for 3 to 5 minutes. The force of this manipulation should be moderate, so it does not to make the patient feeling sore and swollen.

(3) *Moving manipulation*

The doctor, one hand fixing the elbow of the affected limb in place with the thumb on the lateral epicondyle of Humerus and the other four fingers on the inner side of the elbow, the other hand hold the patient's wrist, using the elbow as a pivot, making a flexion and extension movement with the forearm pronating toward the clockwise direction for 10 times. And then, making another flexion and extension movement with the forearm supinating toward the counter-clockwise direction for 10 times. After that, the doctor, carrying the wrist of the affected limb under the arm, keep pulling and extending the elbow for 5 to 7 times.

2.7　Tuina manipulations applied on the wrist and palm

2.7.1　Basic tuina manipulations applied on the wrist and palm

2.7.1.1　Kneading manipulation

The palm kneading manipulation can be used to treat many kinds of diseases. This section contains more pictures to explain the manipulations in further details (Fig.2-212 to Fig.2-220). The tuina manipulations applied on different parts can be used to treat one or several orthopedic diseases of the wrist and palm. For example, the injury of articular disc at the wrist, narrow radial styloid tenosynovitis, the wrist extensor or flexor muscle tendon tenosynovitis, ganglion, distal radial ulnar joint injuries, etc.

2.7.1.2　Pointing manipulation

We can see the pointing manipulation applied on the wrist and palm in Fig.2-221 to Fig.2-224.

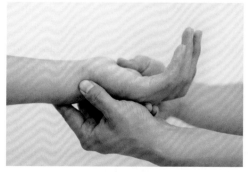 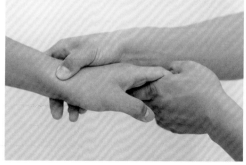

Fig.2-212　Kneading the ulnar side of the wrist　　Fig.2-213　Kneading the radial side of the wrist

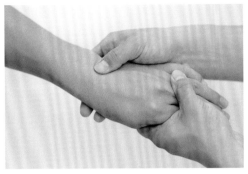

Fig.2-214　Kneading the back side of the wrist

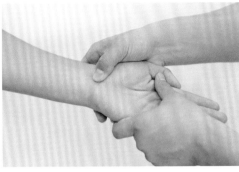

Fig.2-215　Kneading the palm side of the wrist

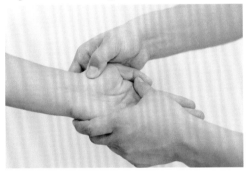

Fig.2-216　Kneading the thenar

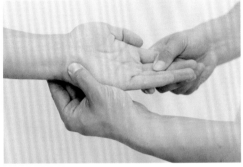

Fig.2-217　Kneading the hypothenar

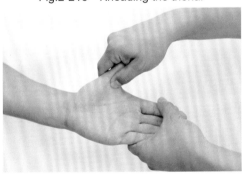

Fig.2-218　Kneading the carpometacarpal joint of thumb

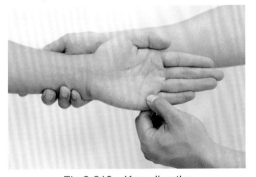

Fig.2-219　Kneading the metacarpophalangeal joint

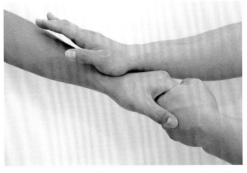

Fig.2-220　Heel of hand kneading manipulation

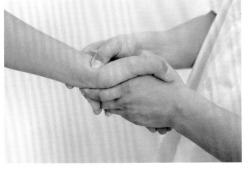

Fig.2-221　Pointing *Yangxi*(LI5)

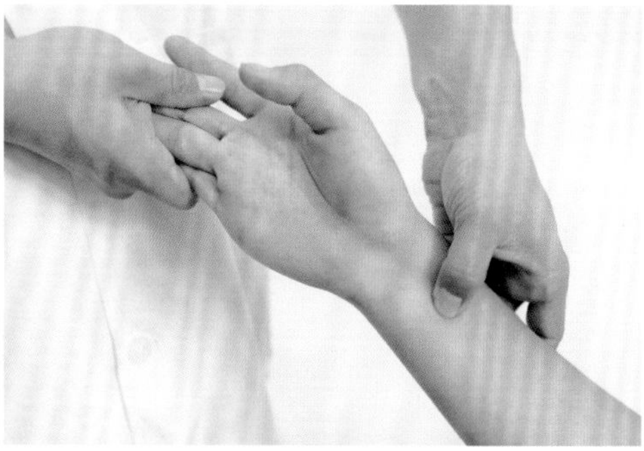

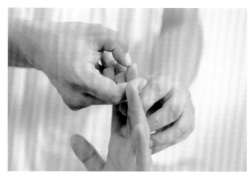

Fig.2-222　Pointing *Neiguan*(PC6)

Fig.2-223　Pointing *Shixuan*(EX-UE11)

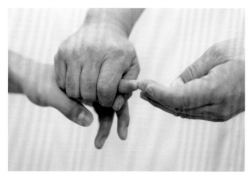

Fig.2-224　Pointing the tip of finger

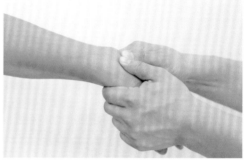

Fig.2-225　Pulling-extending
manipulation on wrist

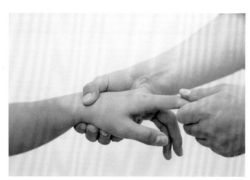

Fig.2-226　The pulling-extending
manipulation on fingers Ⅰ

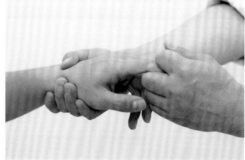

Fig.2-227　The pulling-extending manipulation
on fingers Ⅱ

2.7.1.3　Pulling-extending manipulation

We can see the pulling-extending manipulation applied on the wrist and palm, in Fig.2-225 to Fig.2-228.

2.7.1.4　Smoothing out manipulation

We can see the smoothing out manipulation applied on the wrist and palm in Fig.2-229.

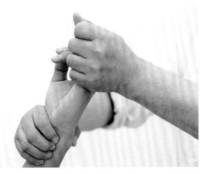

Fig.2-228　The pulling-extending manipulation on fingers III

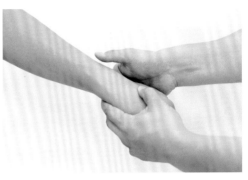

Fig.2-229　Smoothing out manipulation

2.7.1.5　Circle-rotating manipulation with flexion and extension

We can see the circle-rotating manipulation with flexion and extension applied on the wrist and palm in Fig.2-230, Fig.2-231.

2.7.1.6　Rotating manipulation

We can see the rotating manipulation applied on the wrist and palm in Fig.2-232 to Fig.2-234.

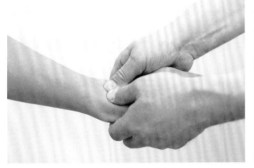

Fig.2-230　Circle-rotating manipulation with flexion and extension I

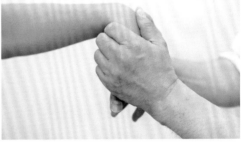

Fig.2-231　Circle-rotating manipulation with flexion and extension II

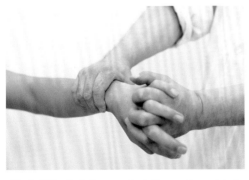

Fig.2-232　Rotating manipulation on the wrist I

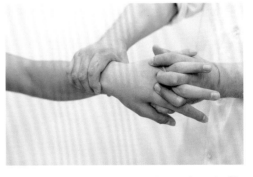

Fig.2-233　Rotating manipulation on the wrist II

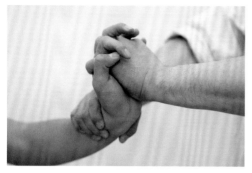

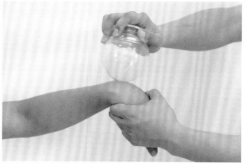

Fig.2-234 Rotating manipulation on the wrist III   Fig.2-235 Breaking up manipulation

2.7.2 Other tuina manipulations applied on the wrist and palm

2.7.2.1 Thecal cyst

(1) *Breaking up manipulation*

If the thecal cyst is located at the back of wrist, the treating technique is: the doctor, holding the patient's hand and flexing the wrist joint to expose the thecal cyst, the other hand break up the thecal cyst with a quick and accurately hit by using the smooth surface of a hard object. (Fig.2-235)

(2) *Crashing manipulation*

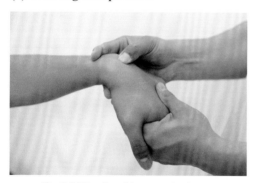

Fig.2-236 Crashing manipulation

If the thecal cyst located at the back of wrist, the treating technique is: the doctor, holding the patient's distal end of the wrist and making the wrist joint flexing to expose the thecal cyst, the thumbs controlling and pressing the thecal cyst, and then, increase the pressing force suddenly to crash the thecal cyst. If the thecal cyst is located at the palmaris side of wrist, then use the manipulation in the opposite direction. (Fig.2-236)

2.7.3 Cases of syndrome differentiation for clinical tuina manipulations

2.7.3.1 Narrow radial styloid tenosynovitis

- Pointing and pressing the following points: *Shousanli*(LI10), *Pianli*(LI6), *Yangxi*(LI5), *Lieque*(LU7), *Hegu*(LI4). Each point should be pressed for 30 seconds.
- Kneading the styloid process region of radius for 5 minutes.

- Smoothing out using the fingers to go up and down with fingers along the abductor pollicis longus tendon and the extensor pollicis brevis tendon for 5 minutes.
- Pulling and extending the wrist joint to make a countertraction, and then regulate the tendon to reduction for 1 to 2 minutes.
- Rubbing on the styloid process region of radius to penetrate the heat into the tissue deeply.

2.8 Tuina manipulations applied on the hip and thigh

2.8.1 Basic tuina manipulations applied on the hip and thigh

2.8.1.1 Rolling manipulation

We can see the rolling manipulation applied on the hip and thigh in Fig.2-237, Fig.2-238.

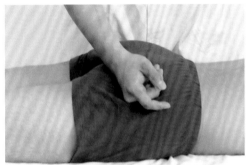 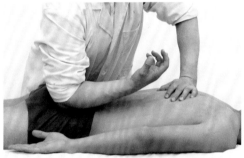

Fig.2-237　Erect rolling manipulation　　　　Fig.2-238　Forearm rolling manipulation

2.8.1.2 Plucking manipulation

We can see the plucking manipulation applied on the hip and thigh in Fig.2-239.

2.8.1.3 Pushing manipulation

We can see the pushing manipulation applied on the hip and thigh in Fig.2-240.

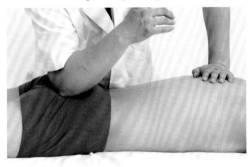 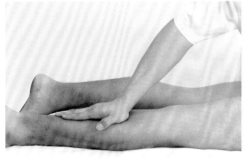

Fig.239　Plucking manipulation　　　　Fig.2-240　Pushing manipulation

2.8.1.4　Grasping manipulation

We can see the grasping manipulation applied on the hip and thigh in Fig.2-241.

2.8.1.5　Pressing manipulation

We can see the pressing manipulation applied on the hip and thigh in Fig.2-242.

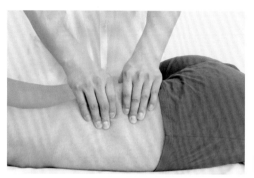

Fig.2-241　Ten-finger grasping manipulation

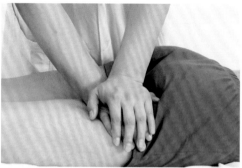

Fig.2-242　Overlapped palm pressing manipulation

2.8.1.6　Pointing manipulation

We can see the pointing manipulation applied on the points *Chengfu*(BL36), *Fengshi*(GB31) in Fig.2-243, Fig.2-244.

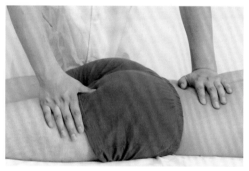

Fig.2-243　Pointing *Chengfu*(BL36)

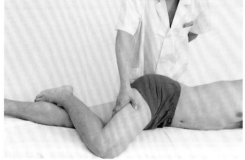

Fig.2-244　Pointing *Fengshi*(GB31)

2.8.1.7　Shaking manipulation

We can see the shaking manipulation on hip joint in Fig.2-245.

2.8.1.8　Kneading manipulation

We can see the kneading manipulation applied on the hip and thigh in Fig.2-246.

2.8.1.9　Moving manipulation

We can see the moving manipulation applied on the hip and thigh in Fig.2-247, Fig.2-248.

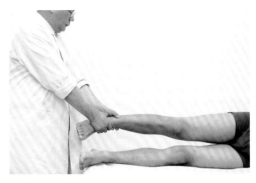

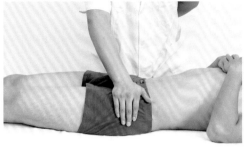

Fig.2-245   The shaking hip joint manipulation.   Fig.2-246   Palm kneading manipulation.

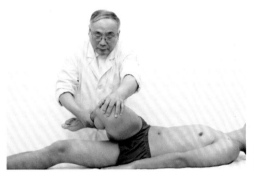

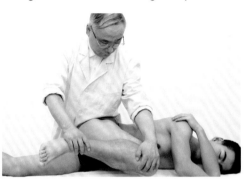

Fig.2-247   Moving manipulation Ⅰ   Fig.2-248   Moving manipulation Ⅱ

2.8.2   Cases of syndrome differentiation for clinical tuina manipulations

2.8.2.1   Piriformis syndrome

(1) *The manipulation used in treating acute phase*

The patient is in the prone position, and the doctor stand beside the affected side of the patient.

- Rolling, pressing and kneading manipulations are worked on the muscles of the hip and the back side of the thigh softly and penetrating the force deeply until the myospasm is relieved. Then use plucking on the piriformis muscle belly with appropriate force.
- Pointing and pressing the following points: *Huantiao*(GB30), *Weizhong*(BL40), *Juliao*(GB29), *Chengfu*(BL36), *Yanglingquan*(GB34) until the patient felt acid and swollen on the points.
- Pushing the piriformis belly from the inner side to the outer side to relax it.

(2) *The manipulation used in treating chronic phase*

- The doctor should operate the rolling, pressing, kneading manipulations worked on the muscles of the hip and lower limb heavily until the myospasm is relieved. Then use plucking on the piriformis muscle belly (the muscle belly may be like band) with appropriate force.
- Pointing and pressing the following points: *Huantiao*(GB30), *Weizhong*(BL40),

Juliao(GB29), *Chengfu*(BL36),etc.

- Moving the hip joint to extension, abduction and extorsion to release adhesion, relieve spasm and reduce pain.
- Rubbing the part to warm the tissues.

2.9 Tuina manipulations applied on the knee and calf

2.9.1 Basic tuina manipulations applied on the knee and calf

2.9.1.1 Kneading manipulation

Because of the complex anatomy of the muscles, tendons, ligaments, and bones around the knee joint, the tuina manipulation can be divided into eight kinds of kneading manipulation according to the direction of tissues. Each kind of manipulation can be used to treat one or several kinds of diseases. So, there are more pictures in this part according to the different locations. (Fig.2-249 to Fig.2-256)

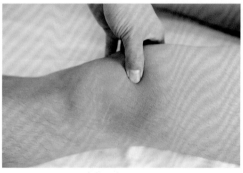

Fig.2-249　Kneading the upper side of the knee joint

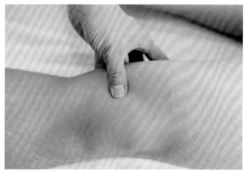

Fig.2-250　Kneading the inner side of the knee joint

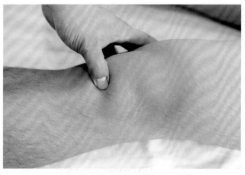

Fig.2-251　Kneading the lower side of the knee joint

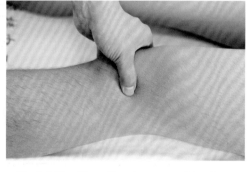

Fig.2-252　Kneading the outer side of the knee joint

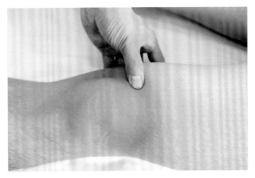

Fig.2-253　Kneading the inner-upper side of the knee joint

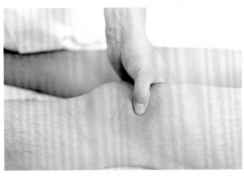

Fig.2-254　Kneading the out-upper side of the knee joint

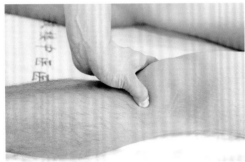

Fig.2-255　Kneading the out-lower side of the knee joint

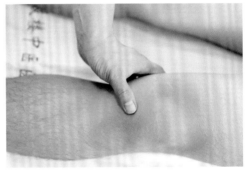

Fig.2-256　Kneading the inner-lower side of the knee joint

2.9.1.2　Pressing and rotating the patella

We can see the pressing and rotating the patella manipulation in Fig.2-257.

2.9.1.3　Pushing and smoothing out the patella

We can see the pushing and smoothing out the patella manipulation in Fig.2-258.

2.9.1.4　Bending and stretching manipulation

The patient takes a supine position with the legs straight. The doctor stands beside the

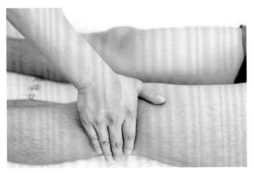

Fig.2-257　Pressing and rotating the patella

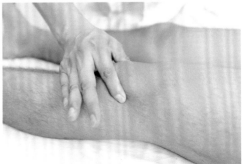

Fig.2-258　Pushing and smoothing out the patella

patient's feet, holding the feet with two hands to bend patient's knee joint first, and then quickly pull the legs straight. Repeat the operation for several times. The pulling strength should be accepted by the patient. (Fig.2-259; Fig.2-260)

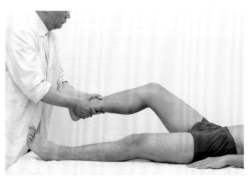

Fig.2-259　Bending and stretching manipulation Ⅰ

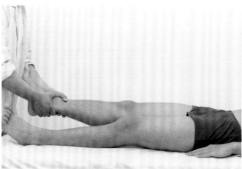

Fig.2-260　Bending and stretching manipulation Ⅱ

2.9.1.5　Grasping manipulation

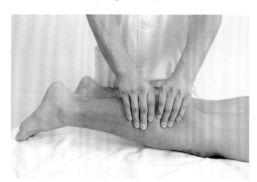

Fig.2-261　The grasping manipulation used on the calf

We can see the grasping manipulation applied on the knee and calf in Fig.2-261.

2.9.1.6　Rotating manipulation

The patient takes a supine position with the hip and knee joint bending to 90°. The operator holds the knee with one hand, and use the other hand to hold the ankle to circular rotate the knee joint. The range of rotating should expand from small to large. The rotating manipulation on the knee joint in prone position can also be used here. (Fig.2-262 to Fig.2-265)

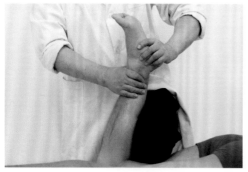

Fig.2-262　Rotating the knee joint manipulation Ⅰ

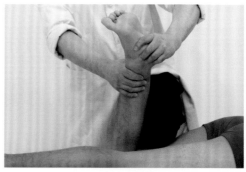

Fig.2-263　Rotating the knee joint manipulation Ⅱ

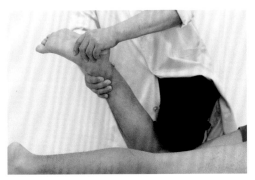

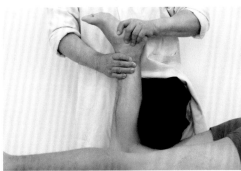

Fig.2-264　Rotating the knee joint
manipulation III

Fig.2-265　Rotating the knee joint
manipulation IV

2.9.1.7　Rolling manipulation

We can see the rolling manipulation applied on the knee and calf in Fig.2-266.

2.9.1.8　Plucking manipulation

We can see the plucking manipulation applied on the point *Weizhong*(BL40) in Fig.2-267.

2.9.1.9　Pointing manipulation

We can see the pointing manipulation applied on the points *Xuehai*(SP10), *Weizhong*(BL40) in Fig.2-268, Fig.2-269.

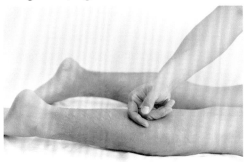

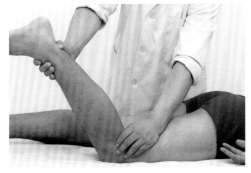

Fig.2-266　Rolling manipulation

Fig.2-267　Plucking the point *Weizhong*(BL40)

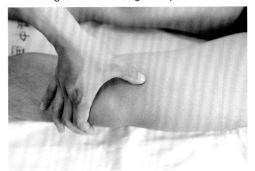

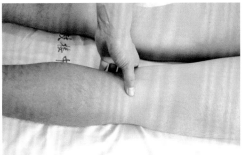

Fig.2-268　Pointing *Xuehai*(SP10)

Fig.2-269　Pointing *Weizhong*(BL40)

2.9.2 Cases of syndrome differentiation for clinical tuina manipulations.

The following diseases should be treated based on the basic tuina manipulations applied to the knee and calf first. And then add or subtract the following manipulations according to the patterns of syndrome.(Attention: Manipulations applied to different parts of the body will be narrated in other sections)

2.9.2.1 Chondromalacia patella

The principles of treatment are dredging collaterals, activating blood circulation to reduce pain.

(1) *Pressing and kneading the patella*

The patient takes a supine position with legs straight and the quadriceps relaxed. The doctor presses the patella to apply the kneading and rotating manipulation with the other hand gently. The force should be controlled so the patient feels no pain or just little pain.

(2) *Pointing and kneading the painful point*

The doctor points and kneads the tissues around the patella and the point *Neixiyan*(EX-LE4) and *Dubi*(ST35)(the two point located in the depression medial and lateral to the patella ligament) with the thumb or index finger and middle finger.

(3) *Pushing and smoothing out the patella*

Clasp the outer edge of the patella with thumb and index finger to do the pushing and smoothing out manipulation up and down.

(4) *Pointing and kneading the points*

Pointing and pressing the points around the knee joint, for example, the points: *Xuehai* (SP10), *Liangqiu*(ST34), *Dubi*(ST35), *Yinlingquan*(SP9), *Yanglingquan*(GB34), *Weiyang* (BL39), *Weizhong*(BL40), etc.

Beside the above manipulations, the rubbing manipulation and the kneading manipulation can be also used here combined with the flexion and extension of the knee joint, the rotating manipulation on the knee joint to improve the clinical therapy effects. The tuina manipulation can be used for once a day or once for every other day. 30 minutes for each time.

2.9.2.2 Osteoarthritis of the knee

The principles of the treatment are activating blood circulation for acesodyne and lubricating the joint.

(1) *Pointing and kneading the painful region*

The patient takes a supine position with the legs straight. The doctor points and kneads the tissues around the knee joint from the inside to the outside and to the round of patella. And then, focus on pointing and kneading the painful region. The force should be controlled so the patient feels no pain.

(2) *Pointing the point to relieve pain*

Pointing and pressing the following points: *Xuehai*(SP10), *Liangqiu*(ST34), *Xiyangguan* (GB33), *Dubi*(ST35), *Yanglingquan*(GB34), *Zusanli*(ST36), *Yinlingquan*(SP9), etc.

(3) *The tuina manipulations on the back side of the knee joint*

The patient turns around to take a prone position. The doctor operates the plucking manipulation on the back side of the knee joint and the thigh.

(4) *Pointing the point to relieve pain*

Pointing and pressing the following points: *Weizhong*(BL40), *Weiyang*(BL39), *Fuxi*(BL38), *Yingu*(KI10), *Heyang*(BL55).

(5) *The rotating manipulation on the knee joint*

(6) *The bending and stretching manipulation on the knee joint*

2.10 Tuina manipulations applied on the foot and ankle

2.10.1 Basic tuina manipulations applied on the foot and ankle

2.10.1.1 Kneading manipulation

We can see the kneading manipulation applied on the foot and ankle in Fig.2-270 to Fig.2-278.

2.10.1.2 Pulling-extending manipulation

We can see the pulling-extending manipulation applied on the foot in Fig.2-279.

2.10.1.3 Rotating manipulation

We can see the rotating manipulation applied on the foot and ankle in Fig.2-280 to Fig.2-282.

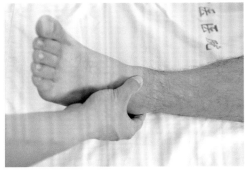 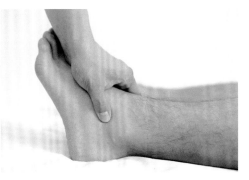

Fig.2-270　Kneading the anterior ankle region　　　Fig.2-271　Kneading the anterior-lateral ankle region

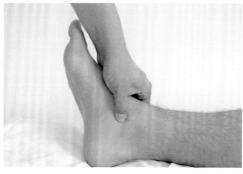

Fig.2-272　Kneading the anterior-medial ankle region

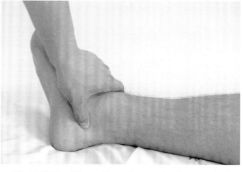

Fig.2-273　Kneading the posterior-medial ankle region

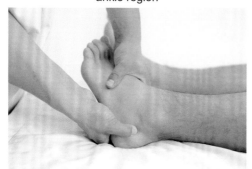

Fig.2-274　Kneading the posterior-lateral ankle region

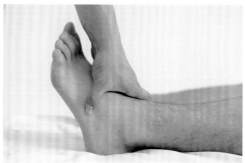

Fig.2-275　Kneading the posterior ankle region

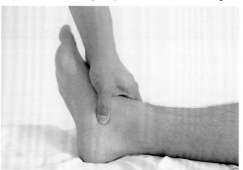

Fig.2-276　Kneading the medial ankle region

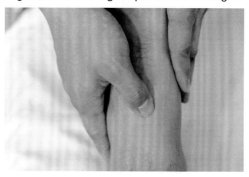

Fig.2-277　Kneading the dorsum of foot

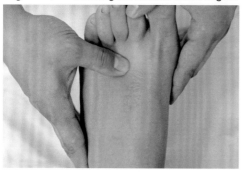

Fig.2-278　Kneading the vola pedis region

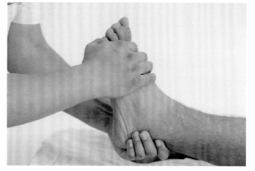

Fig.2-279　Pulling-extending manipulation

2.10.1.4 Grasping manipulation

We can see the grasping manipulation applied on the foot and ankle in Fig.2-283.

2.10.1.5 Smoothing out manipulation

We can see the smoothing out manipulation applied on the foot and ankle in Fig.2-284.

2.10.1.6 Pushing manipulation

We can see the pushing out manipulation applied on the foot and ankle in Fig.2-285.

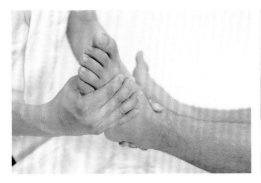

Fig.2-280　Rotating manipulation Ⅰ

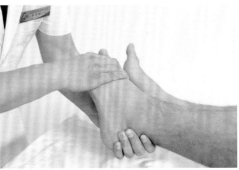

Fig.2-281　Rotating manipulation Ⅱ

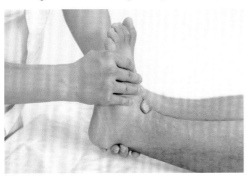

Fig.2-282　Rotating manipulation Ⅲ

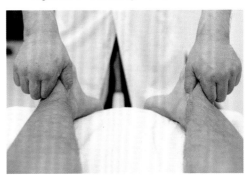

Fig.2-283　Grasping manipulation

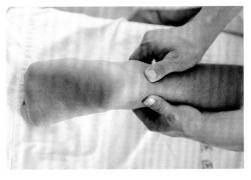

Fig.2-284　Smoothing out manipulation

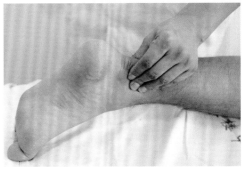

Fig.2-285　Pushing manipulation

2.10.1.7 Pointing manipulation

We can see the pointing manipulation applied on the points *Taichong*(LR3), *Taixi*(KI3), *Kunlun*(BL60), *Sanyinjiao*(SP6) in Fig.2-286 to Fig.2-289.

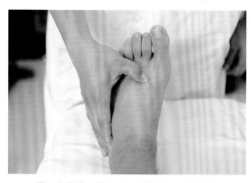

Fig.2-286　Pointing *Taichong*(LR3)

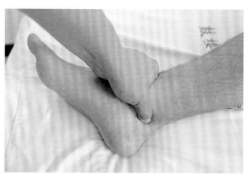

Fig.2-287　Pointing *Taixi*(KI3)

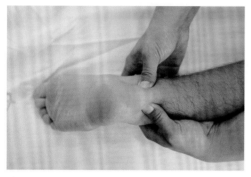

Fig.2-288　Pointing *Kunlun*(BL60) and *Taixi*(KI3) relatively

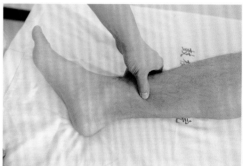

Fig.2-289　Pointing *Sanyinjiao*(SP6)

2.10.2　Other tuina manipulations applied on the foot and ankle

2.10.2.1 Plucking manipulation (see in" calcaneodynia")

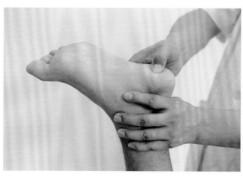

Fig.2-290　Plucking manipulation

We can see the plucking manipulation applied on the foot in Fig.2-290.

2.10.2.2 Pushing manipulation (see in" calcaneodynia")

We can see the pushing manipulation applied on the foot in Fig.2-291.

2.10.2.3 Tapping manipulation (see in"calcaneodynia")

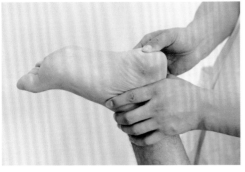
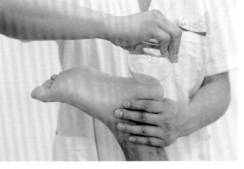

| Fig.2-291 Pushing manipulation | Fig.2-292 Tapping manipulation |

We can see the tapping manipulation applied on the foot in Fig.2-292.

2.10.3 Cases of syndrome differentiation for clinical tuina manipulations

2.10.3.1 Sprain of ankle joint

(1) *Kneading manipulation to eliminate stasis*

The patient sits on the bed with the legs straight. The doctor presses and kneads the affected foot with thumb or thenar eminence. The force should be controlled to knead gently. The manipulation should be operated from the distal end of the limb to the near side, or from the out side of the injured part to the inner side.

(2) *Eliminating swelling to reduce pain*

Apply a small amount of massage cream to the surface the injured region. Operate the thumb circular rubbing manipulation on it, and then, pushing manipulation from the distal end of the limb to the near side to promote the swelling eliminating.

(3) *Lubricating joints*

The doctor, holds the heel of the affected foot with one hand, and applies circular rotating manipulation. The force should be controlled to make the patient feeling no pain. This manipulation is prohibited to be used on a new injury. And it is applied to used on the patient who has sprained the ankle for 2 to 3 weeks and the ankle still pain and the ankle is still in pain with limited range of motion. When rotating the ankle joint, do not use force, especially at the angle in which the patient feels pain, the manipulation should be operated gentle to avoid ligament again.

2.10.3.2 Calcaneodynia

The principle of treatment is pointing to relieve the pain. The manipulations are as follows:

The patient takes a prone position with the legs straight. The doctor presses the Achilles tendon of the affected side with the palm. The thumb over laps with the other thumb and presses on the painful part with force and makes the pushing and plucking manipulation on different direction for 3 to5 minutes, and then using the tapping manipulation. After 2 to 3 times' tuina manipulation treatments, the patient should be satisfied with the effect.

2.11   Manipulations for infantile tuina

In the manipulations for infantile tuina, Professor Cui attached great importance in treating the baby's hand, abdomen, and back. When treating a baby, apply the diagnostic method-inspection method first, followed by the inquiry method, and finishing with listening and smelling. When in inspection, focus mainly on inspecting the fingerprints. The baby skin is thin and delicate, so the collateral vessel can be seen easily. Use these diagnostic techniques for reference. "Differentiate exterior or interior syndrome according to the collateral vessel floating or deep. Judge the deficiency or excess syndrome according to the color of the collateral vessel. Use the fingerprint spectrum, to diagnose the properties and degree of some illness" as the guideline when inspecting the baby's index finger radial sides. Manipulations in hand areas are mainly moving and pushing. For example, pushing zang and fu meridians, moving Bagua, etc. The abdominal wall of baby is thinner and more delicate than the adult, so manipulations on the abdomen have better stimulating and regulating effects on internal organs. The tuina manipulations applied on the abdomen are mainly rubbing and pushing. For example, rubbing the abdomen, and pushing the costal arch with the heel of your hand etc. For the baby's back, the treating points are mainly the shu-back points on the bladder meridian of foot-*taiyang*. They are the points on the back where the qi from zang and fu(every organ) infuse in, and they have special relations with zang and fu. Stimulating them would regulate the internal organs better. The spine pinching, and mainly heel of the hand pushing, manipulations of the back and sacral region should be the basic manipulation techniques. For example, pushing the governor vessel, and pushing the bladder meridian, etc. Among all the manipulations, pushing, kneading and rubbing should be applied most frequently, with the highest frequency, and for the longest time to have the warming and invigorating effect. Nipping and pinching should be applied with firm force, quickly, but less frequently. In addition, Professor Cui Shusheng prefers finger pointing and vibrating manipulation (the finger pointing instead of a needle inserting) in clinical practice, because applying too much acupuncture can damage the baby's yang qi. Professor Cui usually uses his thumbs to press the points and he treats in reference to the nature of the point to deliver the treatment effect. Professor Cui usually select points according to the symptoms, he also attaches importance to partial point selection, for example, selecting from the sacrococcygeal region for treatment of enuresis.

Common used points on infant see Table 2-2.

Table 2-2　Common used points for infantile tuina manipulation

Name of the point	Location	Functions and Indications	Manipulations
Kangong	The transverse line from the medial end to the lateral end of the eyebrow.	Exogenous fever, convulsion, headache, redness and pain of eyes.	Pushing the points respectively from the medial ends of the eyebrows to the lateral ends with both thumbs.
Guiwei(Coccyx)	At the end of the coccyx.	Diarrhea, constipation, rectocele and enuresis.	Kneading the point with the tip of the thumb or the middle finger.
Pijing	On the radial border of the thumb and from the tip to the root.	Diarrhea, dysentery, constipation, loss of appetite, etc.	Circular pushing and pushing along the radical border of the thumb towards the wrist with the infant patient's thumb flexing, this is called reinforcing spleen meridian. Pushing from the opposite direction is called clearing spleen meridian.
Neibagua	The region 2/3 from the center of the palm to the crease at the root of the middle is divided into eight portions.	Cough, asthma due to excessive phlegm, chest oppression, anorexia, abdominal distension, vomiting.	Clockwise moving on the region with the thumb tip is called moving Neibagua or moving Bagua.
Tianheshui (Heaven river water)	Along the midline of forearm from *Zongjin*(great tendon) to *Hongchi*(PC3).	Exogenous fever, tidal fever, internal fever, perspire during sleep, restlessness, etc.	Pushing from the transverse crease of the wrist to that of elbow with the index and middle finger.
Guanyuan(CV4)	On the anterior midline of the lower abdomen, 3 *cun* below the umbilicus.	Secure and tonify the original qi.	Pointing manipulation, pushing manipulation with the heel of palm.
Zhongji(CV3)	On the anterior midline of the lower abdomen, 4 *cun* below the umbilicus.	Tonify the kidney and invigorate yang.	Pointing manipulation, pushing manipulation with the heel of palm.
Shenque(CV8)	In the center of the umbilicus.	Warm and tonify the original yang; fortify the spleen and invigorate the stomach; resuscitate and secure the body.	Pointing manipulation, pushing manipulation with the heel of palm.
Tianshu(ST25)	2 *cun* lateral to the center of the umbilicus.	Regulate the qi and blood circulation; improve the qi activity.	Pointing manipulation, pushing manipulation with the heel of palm.
Qihai(CV6)	On the anterior midline of the lower abdomen, 3 *cun* below the umbilicus.	Develop yang qi.	Pointing manipulation, pushing manipulation with the heel of palm.
Shangwan (CV13)	On the anterior midline of the upper abdomen, 5 *cun* above the umbilicus.	Stomachache, abdominal distension, etc.	Pointing manipulation, pushing manipulation with the heel of palm.
Zhongwan (CV12)	On the anterior midline of the upper abdomen, 4 *cun* above the umbilicus.	Stomachache, abdominal distension, etc.	Pointing manipulation, pushing manipulation with the heel of palm.
Xiawan(CV10)	On the anterior midline of the upper abdomen, 2 *cun* above the umbilicus.	Stomachache, abdominal distension, etc.	Pointing manipulation, pushing manipulation with the heel of palm.

Name of the point	Location	Functions and Indications	Manipulations
Zhangmen (LR13)	On the side of the abdomen, below the free end of the 11th floating rib.	Stomachache, abdominal distension, costalgia, etc.	Pointing manipulation, pushing manipulation with the heel of palm.
Qimen(LR14)	On the chest, directly below the nipple, at the 6th intercostal space, 4 cun lateral to the anterior midline.	Distending pain in the chest and hypochondriac region, diarrhea.	Pointing manipulation, pushing manipulation with the heel of palm.
Huaroumen (ST24)	On the upper abdomen, 1 cun above the center of the umbilicus, 2 cun lateral to the anterior midline of the abdomen.	Stomachache, vomiting, hiccup, borborygmus, indigestion, diarrhea, madness.	Pointing manipulation, pushing manipulation with the heel of palm.
Riyue(GB24)	On the upper abdomen, directly below the nipple, 4 cun lateral to the anterior midline, in the 7th intercostal space.	Jaundice, vomiting, hiccup, etc.	Pointing manipulation, pushing manipulation with the heel of palm
Zusanli(ST36)	On the anteriolateral side of the leg, 3 cun below Dubi (ST35), one finger breadth (middle finger) from the anterior crest of the tibia.	Stomachache, vomiting, abdominal distension, borborygmus, indigestion, atrophy and pain of the legs, etc.	Pointing manipulation.
Taichong(LR3)	On the dorsum of foot, in the depression of the posterior end of the first interosseous metatarsal bones.	Headache, vertigo, hernia, irregular menstruation, enuresis, infantile convulsions, epilepsy, distending pain in the chest and hypochondriac region, etc.	Pointing manipulation.
Shixuan (EX-UE11)	At the tips of the ten fingers, about 0.1 cun distal to the nails, 10 points on left and right fingers.	Clear heat for resuscitation.	Pointing and pinching manipulation.
Yongquan(KI1)	On the sole, in the depression which appears on the anterior part of the sole when the foot is in the plantar flexion, at the junction of the anterior third and posterior two thirds of the line connecting the base of the second and third toes and the heel approximately.	Headache, vertigo, dizziness, dysuria, constipation, etc.	Linear rubbing manipulation, pushing manipulation.
Baliao(BL31-BL34)	On the sacrum, the 8 posterior sacral foramen.	Diseases around the lumbosacral region, lower back pain, sciatica, weakness and paralysis in the lower limbs.	Pushing manipulation.

2.11.1 Basic manipulations for infantile tuina

2.11.1.1 Basic tuina manipulations applied on the abdomen

(1) *Opening the four gates*

The four gates are four points: *Zhangmen*(LR13) is front-mu point of the spleen and one of the eight influential points(*Zang*-organs convergence)(Fig.2-293); *Qimen*(LR14) is front-mu point of the liver(Fig.2-294); *Huaroumen*(ST24) belongs to the stomach meridian of foot-*yangming*(Fig.2-295); *Riyue*(GB24) which is the front-mu point of the gallbladder(Fig.2-296).

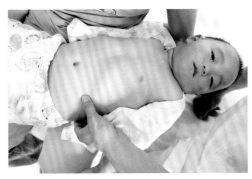

Fig.2-293   Opening the four gates-
Zhangmen(LR13)

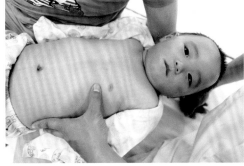

Fig.2-294   Opening the four gates-
Qimen(LR14)

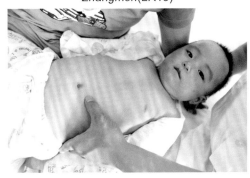

Fig.2-295   Opening the four gates-
Huaroumen(ST24)

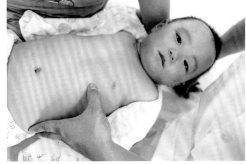

Fig.2-296   Opening the four gates-*Riyue*
(GB24)

(2) *Pointing three wan*

The three wan are three points: *Shangwan*(CV13)(Fig.2-297); *Zhongwan*(CV12)(Fig.2-298); *Xiawan*(CV10)(Fig.2-299).

(3) Tonifying *Shenque*(CV8)(Fig.2-300); Point penetrating *Tianshu*(ST25)(Fig.2-301); Promoting *Qihai*(CV6)(Fig.2-302).

(4) *Scraping the costal arch*

With both hands, use the thumbs pads to press both sides of the chest. Use the circular

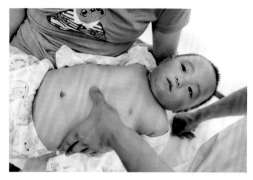

Fig.2-297　Pointing three wan-
Shangwan(CV13)

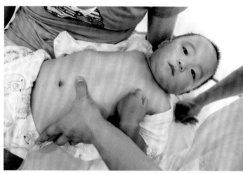

Fig.2-298　Pointing three wan-
Zhongwan(CV12)

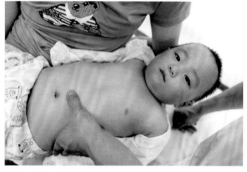

Fig.2-299　Pointing three wan-*Xiawan*(CV10)

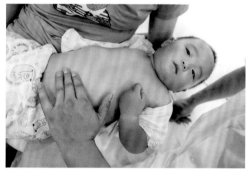

Fig.2-300　Tonifying *Shenque*(CV8)

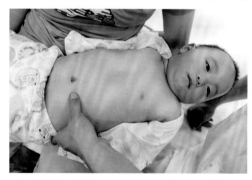

Fig.2-301　Point penetrating *Tianshu*(ST25)

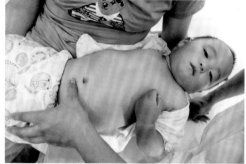

Fig.2-302　Promoting *Qihai*(CV6)

rubbing manipulation along the free end of the 9th rib, the free end of the 10th rib, the free end of the 11th rib, and the free end of the 12th rib. (Fig.2-303)

(5) *Heel of hand pushing manipulation*

Pushing with the heel of hand in these areas in the following order: the costal arch, the upper abdomen, and the lower abdomen. (Fig.2-304 to Fig.2-306)

(6) *Kneading and circular rubbing the abdomen*

With one hand holding the baby on the point *Mingmen*(GV4), knead and use the circular rubbing techniques on the abdomen with the other hand.(Fig.2-307)

(7) *Grasping the Dujiao(sides of abdomen)*

Dujiao is located at 2 *cun* below the umbilicus and 2 *cun* lateral to *Shimen*(CV5). Use the Grasping method on the sides of abdomen with the thumb and index finger. (Fig.2-308)

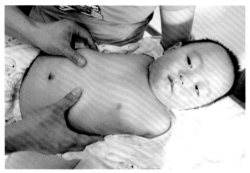

Fig.2-303　Scraping the costal arch

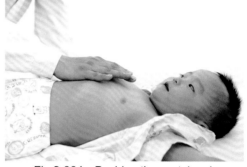

Fig.2-304　Pushing the costal arch

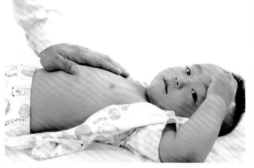

Fig.2-305　Pushing the upper abdomen

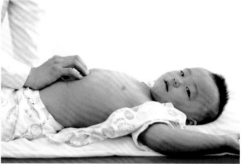

Fig.2-306　Pushing the lower abdomen

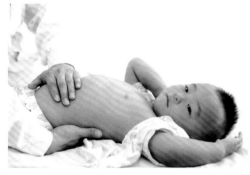

Fig.2-307　Kneading and circular rubbing
the abdomen

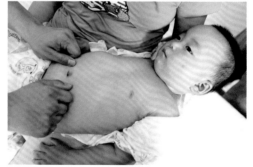

Fig.2-308　Grasping the Dujiao

(8) *Pointing and kneading Zusanli*(ST36)(Fig.2-309)

2.11.1.2　Basic tuina manipulations applied on the back

(1) *Pointing and pressing manipulation along the five lines on the back*

On the Governor Vessel in the middle of the back, use the middle finger, the index finger

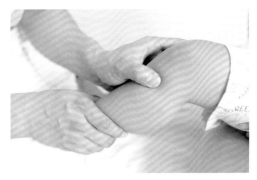

Fig.2-309   Pointing and kneading *Zusanli*(ST36)

and the ring finger of the right hand to manipulate the area with the pointing manipulation. Overlap the left hand over the right hand with close contact to incoprate the pressing technique. On the two branches of the bladder meridian of foot-*taiyang* on each side of the back, use the middle finger and the index finger to use the pointing maneuver (Fig.2-310; Fig.2-311)

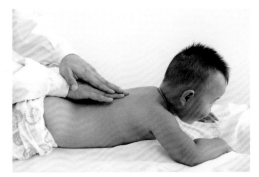

Fig.2-310   Pointing and pressing manipulation along the five lines on the back Ⅰ

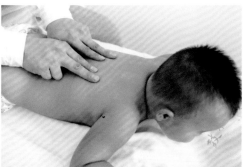

Fig.2-311   Pointing and pressing manipulation along the five lines on the back Ⅱ

(2) *Spine pinching*

Place the sick child in the prone position. Operate the spine pinching manipulation along the bladder meridian of foot-*taiyang* with the four fingers pressing forward and the thumb pinching the skin with both hands (Fig.2-312; Fig.2-313). Use spine pinching manipulation on the five lines on the back two times first, and then pinching three times while lifting to make the skin slightly red. The governor vessel originates from the lower abdomen, descends and emerges at the perineum. It then travels along the interior side of the spinal

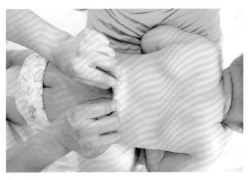

Fig.2-312   Spine pinching Ⅰ

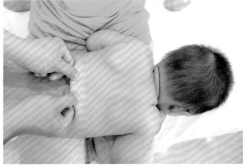

Fig.2-313   Spine pinching Ⅱ

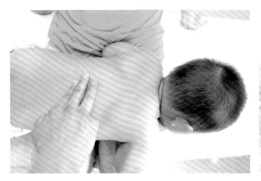

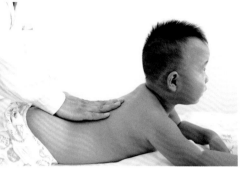

Fig.2-314　Pushing and rubbing the governor vessel

Fig.2-315　Pushing the region *Baliao*(BL31-BL34)

column, entering into the brain, and connects with the Kidney channel. It has the function of governing the yang qi of the whole body and raising it up. The bladder meridian of foot-*taiyang* is located at the both sides of the governor vessel. The back-shu points on the bladder channel can get favorable stimulation with the spine pinching manipulation. By doing so, it can harmonize the functions between organs and treat the relevant organ diseases. So, the spine pinching manipulation on the five lines on the back has the effects of regulating the body function, keeping the balance of yin and yang, invigorate yang qi.

(3) *Pushing and rubbing the governor vessel and bladder meridian*(Fig.2-314)

(4) *Pushing the region Baliao*(BL31-BL34)

The doctor will push with the palm (*Laogong*(PC8)) on the region of *Baliao* (BL31-BL34). The doctor must make sure to touch the palate with the tip of tongue, focusing his/her mind on the point *Laogong*(PC8), exerting pressure from the point *Changqiang*(GV1) to the region *Baliao*(BL31-BL34) for 300 to 500 times(Fig.2-315). This manipulation has the effects of warming and reinforcing the kidney yang, securing the original qi.

(5) *Grasping Jianjing*(GB21)(Fig.2-316)

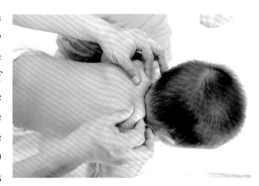

Fig.2-316　Grasping *Jianjing*(GB21)

2.11.2　Other manipulations for infantile tuina

(1) *Grasping and shaking the abdomen*

Grasp the abdomen slowly and gently from up to down along the conception vessel using the slightly shaking manipulation for 10 times (Fig.2-317). For the children who have hard nodule in the lower abdomen, the effect of this manipulation is great. After this manipulation, circular rubbing manipulation should be used to pacify the child.

(2) *Heel of the palm pushing on the points Guanyuan*(CV4) *and Zhongji*(CV3)

This method is used to reinforce the kidney to strengthen the bodies resistance and secure the original qi.(Fig.2-318)

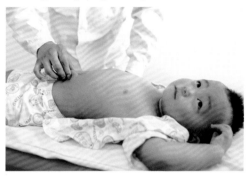 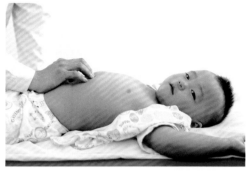

Fig.2-317　Grasping and shaking the abdomen

Fig.2-318　Heel of the palm pushing on the points *Guanyuan*(CV4) and *Zhongji*(CV3)

(3) *Lifting the point Dazhui*(GV14)

The point *Dazhui*(GV14) is located between the spinal processes of the seventh cervical

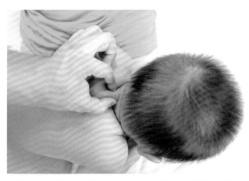

Fig.2-319　Lifting the point *Dazhui*(GV14)

vertebra and the first thoracic vertebra. The lifting method is used with to fingers to make the body sweat, which will release the exterior (Fig.2-319). The point *Dazhui*(GV14) is the crossing point of the six yang meridians and the governor vessel. The yang-heat qi moves in the six yang meridians which all flows into this point. It mixes with the yang qi from governor vessel, and then goes upward to head. Lifting this point with hands has the effects of purging away the heat, removing the exogenous affection and heat out.

(4) *Pushing Qijiegu*(*seven lumbrosacral vertebrae*)

The Qijiegu(seven lumbrosacral vertebrae) is located in the area of the spine from the 4th lumbar vertebrae to the end of the coccyx.

Pushing the lumbrococcygeal vertebrae upward is effective for warming yang to relieve diarrhea. And pushing the lumbrococcygeal vertebrae downward is effective for purging heat to promote defecation. (Fig.2-320)

(5) *Kneading Guiwei*(*coccyx*)

The Guiwei is located at the end of the coccyx. Kneading Guiwei is effective for warming and reinforcing kidney yang, securing original qi. (Fig.2-321)

(6) *Moving Bagua*

With the center of child's palm facing upward, the doctor rubs in a clockwise circular rotation with the index finger and middle finger in the center of child's palm for 49 times. (Fig.2-322)

(7) *Pinching Shixuan*(EX-UE11)

Shixuan(EX-UE11) is located at the tips of the ten fingers, about 0.1 *cun* distal to the nails. In total there are 10 points on the left and right fingers. The doctor pinches the point on the sick child's finger with the thumb and index finger (Fig.2-323). This manipulation has good effect for treating shock, coma, high fever, and infantile syncope. The manipulation of inserting a needle to induce bleeding can also work.

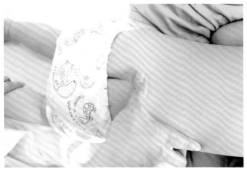

Fig.2-320　Pushing Qijiegu(seven lumbrosacral vertebrae)

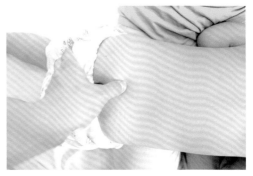

Fig.2-321　Kneading Guiwei(coccyx)

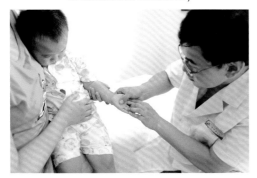

Fig.2-322　Moving Bagua

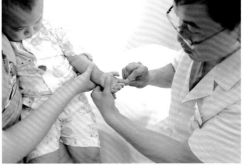

Fig.2-323　Pinching *Shixuan*(EX-UE11)

(8) *Pushing Feijing*

The Feijing is located at the ungual whorl surface of the distal part of the ring finger. The doctor pushes in a circular clockwise rotation with the thumb on the surface of the ring finger 200 times. And then, pushes straight from the finger tip to the transverse crease of the distal interphalangeal joint 200 times (Fig.2-324; Fig.2-325). This manipulation has a good effect for treating infantile cold and fever.

(9) *Reinforcing Pijing*(Fig.2-326)

The Pijing is located on the palmar surface of the distal thumb. Flex the thumb of the child, and then push along the radial border of the thumb towards the wrist. Repeat 200 times. It is effective for treating infantile dyspepsia, diarrhea, vomiting, etc.

(10) *Reinforcing Weijing*(Fig.2-327)

The Weijing is located on the palmar surface of the proximal thumb. Push from the thumb root to the palmar root 200 times. It is effective for treating infantile vomiting, dysphagia.

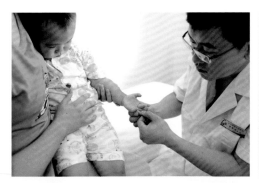 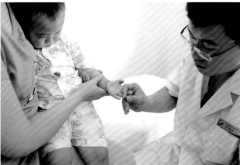

Fig.2-324　Pushing Feijing Ⅰ　　　　Fig.2-325　Pushing Feijing(lung meridian) Ⅱ

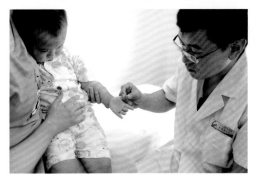 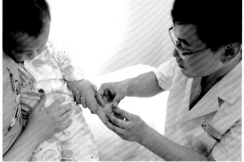

Fig.2-326　Reinforcing Pijing　　　　　Fig.2-327　Reinforcing Weijing

(11) *Kneading Banmen*(*major thenar*)(Fig.2-328)

Banmen is located on the surface of the greater thenar. Kneading the center of the great thenar has the effect of removing pathogenic heat from blood, promoting digestion and eliminating food retention.

(12) *Pushing Sihengwen*(*four transverse creases*)(Fig.2-329)

Pushing Sihengwen means to push the creases from the index finger to the little finger back and forth. It has a good effect for treating infantile malnutrition, abdominal distension and diarrhea.

(13) *Kneading Laogong*(PC8)(Fig.2-330)

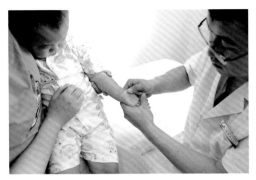

Fig.2-328 Kneading Banmen(major thenar)

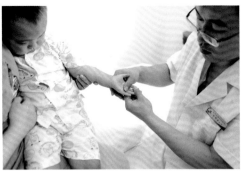

Fig.2-329 Pushing Sihengwen(four transverse creases)

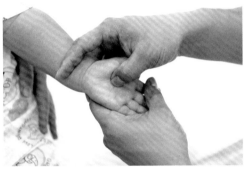

Fig.2-330 Kneading *Laogong*(PC8)

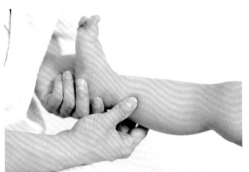

Fig.2-331 Pointing and kneading *Sanyinjiao*(SP6)

(14) *Pointing and kneading Sanyinjiao*(SP6)(Fig.2-331)

(15) *Reinforcing Dachang*(*large intestine*)(Fig.332)

Dachang is located on the radial border of the index finger, from the finger tip to the margin of the web between the index finger and thumb. Pushing from the finger tip to the web margin is considered a reinforcing method, known as reinforcing Dachang. It is effective for astringing the intestine to stop diarrhea. Pushing to the opposite direction is considered as a clearing method, known as clearing Dachang. And it is effective for clearing away heat, eliminating dampness and promoting defecation.

(16) *Clearing Tianheshui*(*heaven river water*)(Fig.2-333)

Push from the transverse crease of the wrist to the elbow(*Quchi*(LI11)) with the thumb with cold water or push from the point *Laogong*(PC8) to the *Quchi*(LI11) with the tip of index finger with cold water. Repeat the manipulation for several times. It has a mild nature of cold, so it is used to treat heat syndromes.

(17) *Pointing Zhongchong*(PC9), *Yongquan*(KI1), *Taichong*((LR3)(Fig.2-334 to Fig.2-336)

(18) *Pushing Sanguan*(*triple pass*)(Fig.2-337)

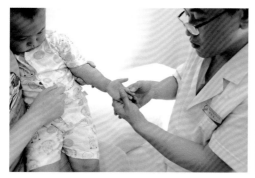

Fig.2-332 Reinforcing Dachang(large intestine)

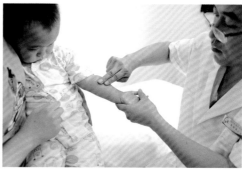

Fig.2-333 Clearing Tianheshui(heaven river water)

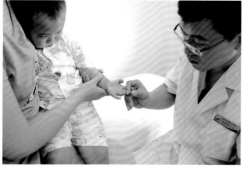

Fig.2-334 Pointing *Zhongchong*(PC9)

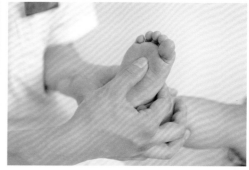

Fig.2-335 Pointing *Yongquan*(KI1)

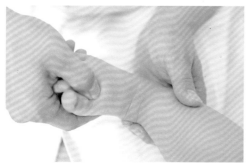

Fig.2-336 Pointing *Taichong*(LR3).

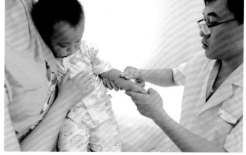

Fig.2-337 Pushing Sanguan(triple pass)

Sanguan is located on the radial aspect of the forearm on the line between *Yangxi*(LI5) and *Quchi*(LI11). Pushing with the bellies of the index and middle fingers or the radial side of the thumb from the point *Yangxi*(LI5) which is located on the radial side of the wrist to the point *Quchi*(LI11) located on the radial side of the elbow. It has good effects for treating infantile cold, deficiency type diarrhea and abdominal pain.

(19) *Opening Tianmen (the heaven gate)*(Fig.2-338)

The infantile patient lies down in a supine position. The doctor sits in front of child's head with each hand located at each side of the head. Pushing down with the pads of both thumbs alternately, from the point *Yintang*(GV29) to the point *Shenting*(GV24) straight upward. Repeat the manipulation 100 times.

(20) *Scalping the eyebrow arc*(Fig.2-339)

The doctor uses the radial side of the thumbs to locate the midpoint between the two eyebrows. From there, push the eyebrow arc respectively to the lateral ends of the eyebrows. Repeat the manipulation 100 times.

(21) *Separating yin and yang*(Fig.2-340)

The doctor uses the pad of both thumbs on the infantile patient's forehead, taking the line from the point *Yintang*(GV29) to the point *Shenting*(GV24) as the midline, separately pushing from the midline to the lateral sides. Repeat the manipulation 100 times.

(22) *Kneading the point Baihui*(GV20)(Fig.2-341)

Because of the infantile fontanel is not closed, the doctor should knead the point *Baihui*(GV20) gently and softly for 1 to 2 minutes.

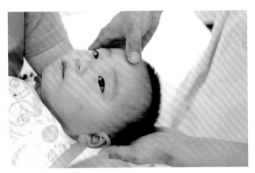
Fig.2-338　Opening Tianmen(the heaven gate)

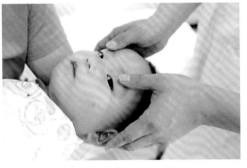
Fig.2-339　Scalping the eyebrow arc

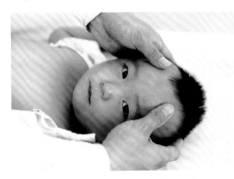
Fig.2-340　Separating yin and yang

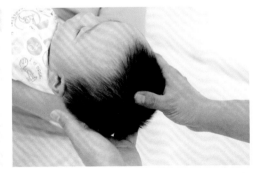
Fig.2-341　Kneading the point *Baihui*(GV20)

2.11.3　Cases of syndrome differentiation for clinical tuina manipulations

2.11.3.1　Infantile enuresis

Treatment principle: warming and tonifying spleen and kidney, securing original qi.

- Basic tuina manipulations applied on the back.
- Pushing the *Baliao*(BL31-BL34), Guiwei(coccyx) from down to up with the heel of palm.
- Pushing the points *Guanyuan*(CV4), *Zhongji*(CV3)(belonging to the conception vessel, located below the umbilicus 3 *cun* and 4 *cun*) with the heel of palm.

2.11.3.2   Infantile common cold

- Basic tuina manipulations:
  - — Moving Bagua.
  - — Pinching *Shixuan*(EX-UE11).
  - — Pushing Feijing(lung meridian).
- For the infantile patient who has cold and has dyspepsia caused by excessive eating or improper diet, the following manipulations should be used beside the basic tuina manipulation.
  - — The infantile patient takes a prone position. The doctor presses the points on the bladder meridian from top to down for 3 to 5 times.
  - — With the four fingers pressing ahead and the thumb supporting behind, do the spine pinching manipulation along the governor vessel from down to up for 5 times. In the first 3 rounds, the manipulation should be operated slightly and quickly. In the last 2 rounds, pinching 3 times and then lifting once from the Qijiegu(coccyx).
  - — The infantile patient takes a supine position. The doctor rubs the patient's abdomen in a clockwise circular 49 times.
  - — Opening the four gate: pointing and pressing the four points *Zhangmen*(LR13), *Qimen*(LR14), *Huaroumen*(ST24), *Riyue*(GB24); Pointing three wan: *Shangwan* (CV13), *Zhongwan*(CV12), *Xiawan*(CV10). Repeat each manipulation for 3 to 5 times.
- For the infantile patient who has a cold and is also afraid, the following manipulations should be used besides the basic tuina manipulation.
  - — Opening Tianmen(the heaven gate).
  - — Scalping the eyebrow arc.
  - — Separating yin and yang.
  - — Kneading the point *Baihui*(GV20).
- For the infantile patient who has a cold and also has fever, the following manipulations should be used besides the basic tuina manipulation.
  - — Spine pinching manipulation.
  - — Lifting the point *Dazhui*(GV14).
  - — Pushing the eyebrow arc.

— Clearing Tianheshui(heaven river water).

For the infantile patient with a persistent fever, the points: *Zhongchong*(PC9), *Yongquan* (KI1), *Taichong*(LR3) should be pointed.

2.11.3.3 Infantile anorexia

- Basic tuina manipulations applied on the back.
- Circular rubbing manipulation on the abdomen.
- Reinforcing Pijing(spleen meridian), Reinforcing Weijing(stomach meridian), Moving Neibagua, Kneading Banmen(major thenar), Pushing Sihengwen(four transverse creases). The manipulations of Reinforcing Pijing(spleen meridian) and Reinforcing Weijing(stomach meridian) have the effects of fortifying the spleen and harmonizing the stomach, promoting the function of spleen and stomach. The manipulations of Moving Neibagua, Kneading Banmen(major thenar), Pushing Sihengwen(four transverse creases) have the effects of regulating qi moving, keeping balance of yin and yang, assisting the function of spleen and stomach.
- For the patient who has undigested food in stool, the manipulations Moving Neibagua and kneading *Zusanli*(ST36) should be used. For the infantile patients who are crying and screaming, the point *Laogong*(PC8), *Sanyinjiao*(SP6) should be kneaded alternatively for 50 times.

2.11.3.4 Infantile diarrhea

- Basic tuina manipulations applied on the abdomen.
- For the infantile patient who has diarrhea caused by excessive eating or improper diet, the following manipulations should be used besides the basic tuina manipulation. Reinforcing Pijing(spleen meridian), Kneading Guiwei(coccyx). Reinforcing Pijing(spleen meridian) could fortify the spleen, help digest the food and relieving dyspepsia. Kneading Guiwei(coccyx) could regulate intestinal functions to stop diarrhea.
- For the infantile patient who has diarrhea caused by spleen deficiency.

Reinforcing Pijing(spleen meridian), Reinforcing Dachang(large intestine), Pushing Qijiegu(seven lumbrosacral vertebrae), Kneading Guiwei(coccyx) should be used. The manipulations of Reinforcing Pijing(spleen meridian) and Reinforcing Dachang(large intestine) could fortify spleen to supplement qi, and secure the intestine. The manipulations of Pushing Qijiegu(seven lumbrosacral vertebrae) and Kneading Guiwei(coccyx) could warm yang to stop diarrhea.

2.11.3.5 Infantile constipation

- Basic tuina manipulation:
  — Circular rubbing the abdomen.

— Pointing the three wan.

— Grasping and shaking the abdomen.

• For constipation of excess type

Clearing Tianheshui (heaven river water), Clearing Dachang(large intestine), Pushing Qijiegu (seven lumbrosacral vertebrae), Kneading Guiwei(coccyx) should be used. The manipulations of Clearing Tianheshui(heaven river water) and Clearing Dachang(large intestine) could eliminate the heat in stomach and intestine. The manipulations of Pushing Qijiegu(seven lumbrosacral vertebrae) and Kneading Guiwei(coccyx) could clear the hollow viscera to assist bowel movement.

• For the constipation of deficiency type

Reinforcing Pijing, Pushing Feijing, Pushing Sanguan(triple pass), Kneading the point *Zusanli*(ST36), Pushing Qijiegu(seven lumbrosacral vertebrae) should be used. The lung dominates the movement of qi and the spleen contains blood. So, kneading to reinforcing lung and spleen meridian could tonify blood and invigorate qi; the Sanguan could enrich blood and qi to treat several kinds of diseases of deficiency. The point *Zusanli*(ST45) could fortify spleen and harmonize stomach, regulate qi movement in the abdomen. The manipulation of Pushing Qijiegu(seven lumbrosacral vertebrae) could clear the hollow viscera to assist bowel movement.

2.11.3.6　Infantile myogenic torticollis

(1) *Relax the affected part*

The infantile patient takes a supine position. The doctor sits in front of the child's head holding the occiput of the patient with one hand to uplift the head to a hyperextended position. Apply kneading manipulation on the sternocleidomastoid muscle gently and softly with the whorl surface of the thumb. Treat the healthy side first and then the affected side later. Repeat the manipulation on each side for 8 to 10 times. (Fig.2-342)

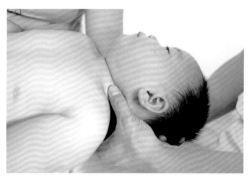

Fig.2-342　Kneading manipulation

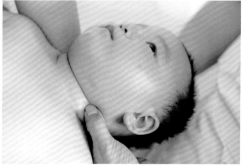

Fig.2-343　Plucking manipulation

(2) *Plucking the tendon to dissolve lumps*

The doctor applies the thumb plucking manipulation along the sternocleidomastoid muscle. The manipulation should be performed gently from the distal end to the affected area. When operating on the affected area, the force should be increased to pluck 3 to 5 times with the pad of the thumb. Use the same operation on the beginning and ending points of the sternocleidomastoid muscle. Repeat the manipulation for 8 to 10 times. (Fig.2-343)

(3) *Pulling manipulation*

The infantile patient takes a supine position. The doctor sits in front of the child's head. While holding the occiput of the patient with one hand, grasp the patient's lower jaw with the other hand. Pull the patient's head gradually toward the normal side to make the head flex to the normal side and then the face rotates to the affected side, so as to correct the torticollis. (Fig.2-344)

(4) *Straight pushing manipulation for relaxing*

The infant patient takes a prone position or is held by the parent. The doctor, holding the patient's head to flex towards the normal side with one hand, applies the straight pushing manipulation on the sternocleidomastoid muscle of the affected side with the other hand for 8 to 10 times. (Fig.2-345)

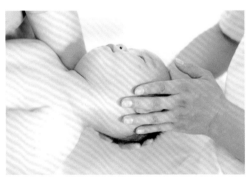
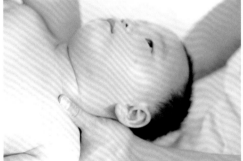

Fig.2-344　Flexing the neck　　Fig.2-345　Straight pushing manipulation

2.11.3.7　Infantile subluxation of radial head

On the the left side for example: the parent holds the child in a sitting position, while the doctor stands at the opposite side. The doctor puts his right thumb on the lateral side of the humeral head with the hand holding the child's elbow, while he holds the wrists with the left hand. Bend the elbow and create internal rotation first, and then unbend and pull the arm, after that, externally rotate the affected elbow, and push upward with the thumb of the right hand at the same time. The cracking sound can be heard to show the reduction successful. After the reduction, the child should stretch out the hand to reach for objects in order to show recovery. (Fig.2-346 to Fig.2-349)

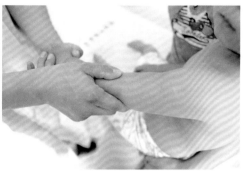

Fig.2-346　Kneading manipulation

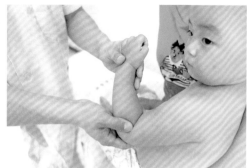

Fig.2-347　Bending and internal rotating the elbow

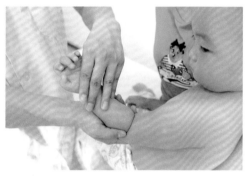

Fig.2-348　Stretching the arm and pulling

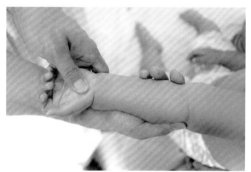

Fig.2-349　Pushing upward with external rotating

2.11.3.8　Infantile transient synovitis of the hip

(1) *Relax the affected part*

The infantile patient takes a supine position. Relax the muscles around the hip joint for 3 to 5 minutes with kneading, rolling, plucking and pushing manipulation. Focus on relaxing the femoral lateral rectus muscle. (Fig.2-350)

(2) *Focus on pointing point*

Find the most painful point on the partial area. Focus on pointing into it for 2 to 3 minutes.

(3) *Reduction manipulation*

On the left side for example: The infant patient takes supine position, the doctor stands at the patient's left side and face towards the patient, holding the affected limb by the ankle with his right hand, while securing the knee joint with the left hand. Gently bend the limb inward to the lowest position trying to keep close to the abdomen. While bending inward, give a firm outward pulling manipulation, repeat 3 times(Fig.2-351 to Fig.2-353). Generally after 2 to 3 times, the patient will be recovered.

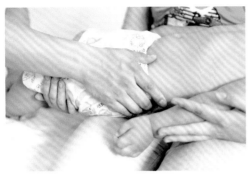

Fig.2-350 Relax the affected part

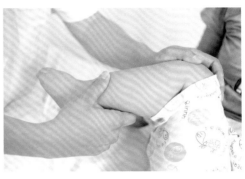

Fig.2-351 Bending the hip and knee joint

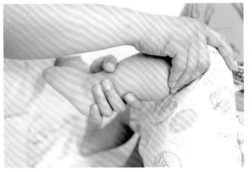

Fig.2-352 Touching abdomen with
internal rotating

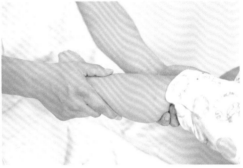

Fig.2-353 Stretching straight with
internal rotating

[Chapter 3]

Exercises for Manipulation Practice

3.1 Eighteen Exercises for practice

The Eighteen Exercises for practice is a way of body-buildup in order to prevent and treat pains in the neck, shoulder, lower back and legs in combination with medical and sports sciences, which is gradually established on the basis of traditional Chinese medicine such as Daoyin, Wuqinxi and Baduanjin and heritage of Wushu. It is particularly useful for working grown-ups who keep in a similar stance for long, additionally for moderately aged and elderly individuals.

3.1.1 Exercises for the prevention and treatment of the pain on the neck and shoulder

The training exercises include head and shoulder girdle movements, which can improve and recover the activity function of the neck, shoulder and fingers. It can also smooth the liver and promote circulation of qi. This exercise also helps with the digestion, and regulates cerebral function.

3.1.1.1 Strength-competition between muscles on the neck and nape

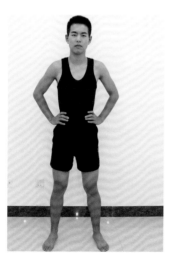

Fig.3-1

Stand upright with legs apart slightly wider than a shoulder width. Put both hands upon the hip with thumbs backward. (Fig.3-1)

(1) Turn the face to the left of the body maximally with eyes looking the left. (Fig.3-2)

(2) Return to the relaxing position.

(3) Turn the face to the right of the body maximally with

eyes looking the right. (Fig.3-3)

(4) Return to the commencing position.

(5) Raise the head to look up.(Fig.3-4)

(6) Return to the commencing position.

(7) Lower the head to look down. (Fig.3-5)

(8) Return to the commencing position.

【Frequency】

2-4 sets of 8 beats.

【Arrival of qi】

You will feel soreness and swelling in the cervical muscles.

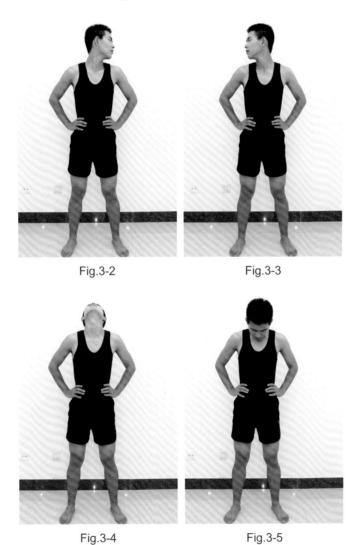

Fig.3-2   Fig.3-3

Fig.3-4   Fig.3-5

3.1.1.2 Drawing the bow on the left and right

Stand upright with legs apart slightly wider than shoulder width. *Hukou* (the part between thumb and the four fingers) of both hands are raised oppositely into round about 30 cm off the face with the palms forward and eyes looking straight ahead. (Fig.3-6)

(1) Both hands are drawn back to the body sides gently making fists, the plane of the fists straight forward, with elbow naturally placed. Turn face to the left and the eyes are looking at distant place to the left. (Fig.3-7)

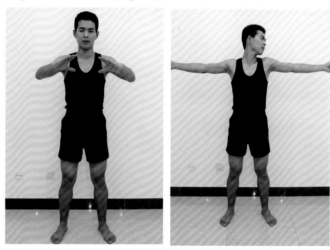

Fig.3-6   Fig.3-7

(2) Return to the commencing position.

(3) and (4) are the same with(1) and (2) but face turning to the right.

【Frequency】

2-4 sets of 8 beats.

【Arrival of qi】

When lifting the chest and looking at distant place, there will be a feeling of soreness and swelling in the neck, shoulders and back muscles. The feelings radiate to the muscle group in both arms, and there will be a comfortable feeling in the chest.

3.1.1.3 Stretching arms upward

Stand upright with legs apart and flex elbows at the sides of the body with hands gently making fists higher than the shoulder to keep the palms forward. (Fig3-8)

(1) Loosen both fists and raise the arms at the same time with the palms forward, head up and eyes focusing on fingers on the affected side. (Fig.3-9)

(2) Return to the commencing position.

(3) and (4) are the same with (1) and (2) but in the opposite direction. (Fig.3-10)

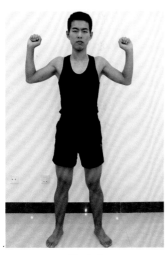 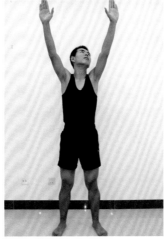 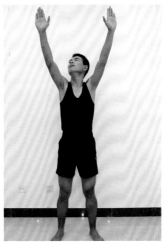

| Fig.3-8 | Fig.3-9 | Fig.3-10 |

【Frequency】

2-4 sets of 8 beats.

【Arrival of qi】

When looking up at the fingers, there will be a feeling of soreness and swelling in the neck and shoulders. When abdomen in and chest out, there will be a feeling of soreness and swelling in the lower back.

3.1.1.4 Chest-open exercise

Stand upright with legs apart and both hands are crossed before the belly with the back of hands in front.(Fig.3-11)

(1) Both arms are raised up crossed with the eyes focusing on the back of the hands. (Fig.3-12)

(2) Both arms fall along the sides of the body in arc trace with palms turning over and return to commencing position. (Fig.3-13)

(3) and (4) are the same with (1) and (2).

【Frequency】

2-4 sets of 8 beats.

【Arrival of qi】

When raising the two arms, you will feel soreness and swelling in the neck, shoulder and lower back.

3.1.1.5 Open arms like birds flying

Stand upright with legs apart and both hands fall relaxed.

(1) The arms are opened behind the body like bird spreading the wings with the hands

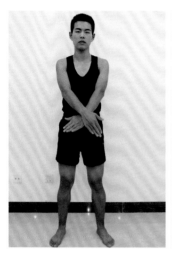
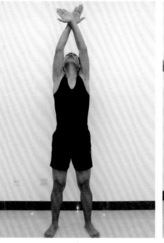
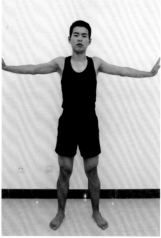

| Fig.3-11 | Fig.3-12 | Fig.3-13 |

drooping and the back of the hands facing each other and the eyes are looking at the left elbow. (Fig.3-14)

(2) When the arms are falling, the hands are turned over in front of the face with palms erected and opposite and slowly fall to return to the commencing position. (Fig.3-15)

(3) and (4) are the same with (1) and (2) but eyes focusing on right elbow. (Fig.3-16)

【Frequency】

2-4 sets of 8 beats.

【Arrival of qi】

You will feel soreness and swelling in the shoulder and both sides of the chest.

3.1.1.6   Lifting with strong arm

Stand upright with legs apart and hands fall naturally.

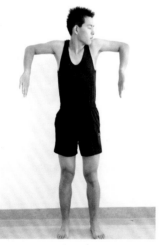
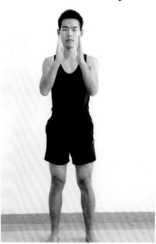
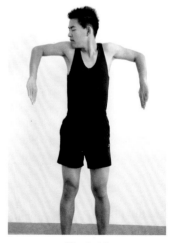

| Fig.3-14 | Fig.3-15 | Fig.3-16 |

(1) The left arm is raised up along the side of the body with palm up and eyes looking at the back of the hand, meanwhile the right arm is stretched backward, flex the elbow toward the low back and then the back of hand is tightly put on it. (Fig.3-17)

(2) The left hand fall along the side of the body and then placed above the right wrist against the low back. (Fig.3-18)

(3) and (4) are the same with (1) and (2) but for the right arm.

【Frequency】

2-4 sets of 8 beats.

【Arrival of qi】

When the arm is raising up with palm up, you will feel soreness and swelling in the neck and shoulder at the same side and will feel comfortable in the chest.

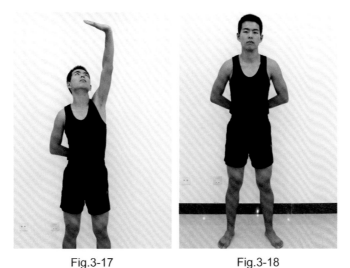

Fig.3-17   Fig.3-18

3.1.2　Exercises for prevention and treatment of the pain on the lower back

The training exercises include low back and hip movements. The actions make joints lubricating and enhance the muscle strength of low back and abdomen. In addition, it is helpful to correct spinal scoliosis, regulate spleen and stomach, eliminate chest and abdominal fullness, solidify the kidney and nourish sperm, etc.

3.1.2.1　Holding the heaven with arms

Stand upright with legs apart and hands crossed upon the upper abdomen and palms up.(Fig.3-19)

(1) Raise both arms up beneath the jaw. Turn and raise the palms over the head with chin up, chest out and palms up. (Fig.3-20; Fig.3-21)

(2) The arms pull the upper part of the body bending to the left once. (Fig.3-22)

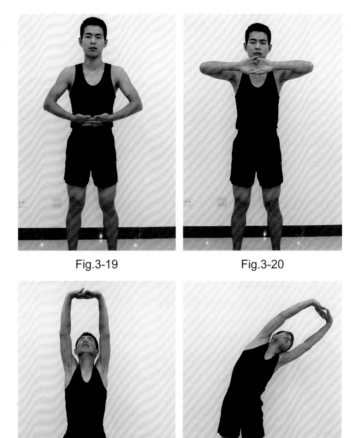

Fig.3-19 Fig.3-20

Fig.3-21 Fig.3-22

(3) Bend once again.

(4) The arms fall along the sides of the body to the commencing position.

(5)-(8) Are the same with (1)-(4) but in the opposite direction.

【Frequency】

2-4 sets of 8 beats.

【Arrival of qi】

You will feel soreness and swelling in the cervical and lumbar muscles. And the feeling can spread to the shoulders, arms and fingers.

3.1.2.2 Pushing palm with waist turning

Stand upright with legs apart and hands clenching upon the hip. (Fig.3-23)

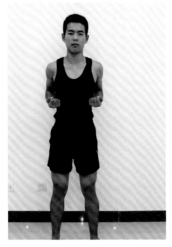
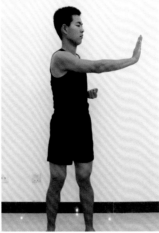

Fig.3-23   Fig.3-24

(1) Push the right hand forward with the palm erected and upward, and meanwhile the upper part of the body turn to the left with the eyes looking at the left, left elbow raised to the far left and the left arm paralleled to the right one.(Fig.3-24)

(2) Turn to the commencing position.

(3) and (4) are the same with (1) and (2) but in the opposite direction.

【Frequency】

2-4 sets of 8 beats.

【Arrival of qi】

Feel soreness and swelling in the cervical and lumbar muscles and shoulder.

【Application】

It is applicable for soft tissue strain in neck, shoulder, back and low back, such as neck and low back pain with numb arms, muscle atrophy, etc.

3.1.2.3 Rotation with hands on hips

Stand upright with legs apart, and put both hands upon the hip with thumbs forward.

(1)-(4) Push the pelvis to circle clockwise once by both hands. (Fig.3-25)

(5)-(8) are the same with (1)-(4) but circle anticlockwise once.

【Frequency】

2-4 sets of 8 beats.

【Arrival of qi】

You will feel distinctly soreness and swelling in the lower

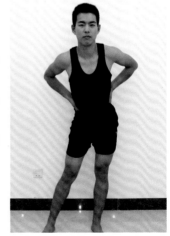

Fig.3-25

back.

3.1.2.4 Bending down with arms spread

Stand upright with legs apart, and the hands crossing before abdomen with palms inward. (Fig.3-26)

(1) Raise the arms forward and up with chin in, chest out and abdomen in, eyes looking at the back of the hands. (Fig.3-27)

(2) The arms fall along the sides of the body to horizon line with palms up. (Fig.3-28)

(3) Turn the palms down. And meanwhile the upper part of the body bends forward with low back straight.

(4) The arms cross before the body. (Fig.3-29)

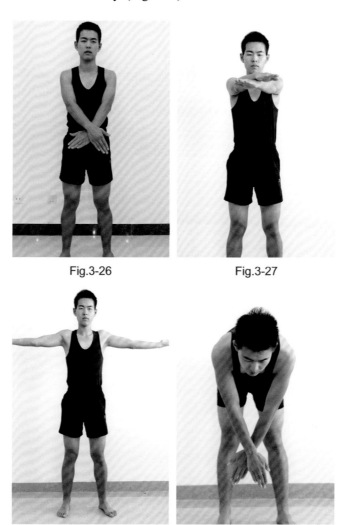

Fig.3-26   Fig.3-27

Fig.3-28   Fig.3-29

(5)-(8) are the same with (1)-(4) and return to commencing position at last beat.

【Frequency】

2-4 sets of 8 beats.

【Arrival of qi】

You will feel soreness and swelling when raising arms and looking at the back of the hands, and will feel soreness and swelling in leg muscles when the hands touch the ground.

3.1.2.5 Inserting palm with lunges position

Stand up right with legs apart for a large step with hands clenching upon hips. (Fig.3-30) (1) Turn the upper part of the body to the left in left bow step, and meanwhile the right fist open to show the palm and thrust the palm forward and up with thumb paralleled to the top of the head.(Fig.3-31)

(2) Return to the commencing position.

(3) and (4) are the same with (1) and (2) but in the opposite direction.

【Frequency】

2-4 sets of 8 beats.

【Arrival of qi】

You will feel soreness and swelling in the lower back and legs.

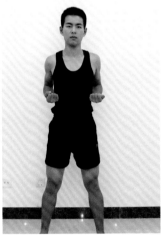 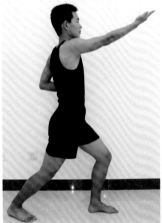

Fig.3-30   Fig.3-31

3.1.2.6 Climbing feet with hands

Stand with hands falling relaxed.

(1) Fingers cross before the upper abdomen with palms up and turn over the palms when passing the face to palms up with eyes looking at the back of the hands(Fig.3-32)

(2) The upper part of the body bends with low back straight.

(3) Push the palms at the insteps. (Fig.3-33)

(4) Return to the commencing position.

(5)-(8) are the same to (1)-(4).

【Frequency】

2-4 sets of 8 beats.

【Arrival of qi】

You will feel soreness and swelling in the neck and lower back when raising the arms, and feel soreness and swelling in the lower back and legs when lower back bend with palms arriving at insteps.

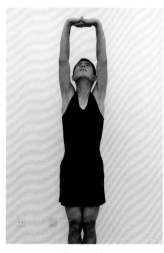 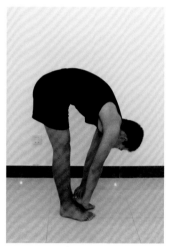

Fig.3-32   Fig.3-33

3.1.3   Exercises for prevention and treatment of the pain on the hip and legs

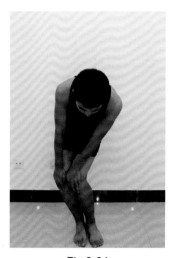

The training exercises include hip and legs movement. The movements of hip, knee and ankle enhance the muscle strength in low back, abdomen and legs and correct spinal and pelvic malformation, etc.

3.1.3.1   Turning knees left and right

The upper part of the body bends with hands over the knees and eyes looking forward and down.

(1) The legs bend and make a circle clockwise once with legs straight when circling to the back. (Fig.3-34)

(2) Return to the commencing position.

(3) and (4) are the same with (1) and (2).

(5)-(8) are the same with (1)-(4) but in opposite direction at the second set of 8 beats.

Fig.3-34

2-4 sets of 8 beats.

【Arrival of qi】

You will feel soreness and swelling in knees and ankles when circling the knees.

3.1.3.2 Turning body in crouching step

Stand upright with legs apart for a large step, and put both hands upon the hips with thumbs backward.(Fig.3-35)

(1) The left leg turns to crouch step with the upper part of the body turn left for 45°. (Fig.3-36)

(2) Return to the commencing position.

(3) and (4) are the same with (1) and (2) but in the opposite direction.

【Frequency】

2-4 sets of 8 beats.

【Arrival of qi】

You will feel soreness and swelling in adductor muscles of the unbent leg and in quadriceps femoris of the bent leg in crouch step.

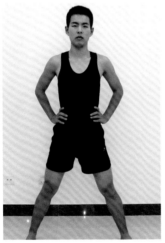 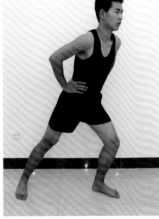

Fig.3-35   Fig.3-36

3.1.3.3 Stretching legs with crouching step

Stand with hands falling relaxed.

(1) The upper part of the body bends with hands over the knees and keep legs straight.

(2) Make a full squat with hands over the knees and fingertips facing each other.

(3) Put both hands on the back of each feet and then straighten the legs(Fig.3-37).

(4) Return to the commencing position; (5)-(8) are the same to (1)-(4).

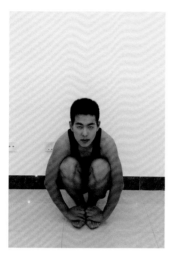

Fig.3-37

【Frequency】

2-4 sets of 8 beats.

【Arrival of qi】

You will feel soreness and swelling in the anterior muscles of thigh during full squat and in the posterior muscles of thigh and calf when straighten the legs and it aggravates to put both hands on the back of each feet.

3.1.3.4 Supporting knee and holding palm

Stand upright with legs apart wider than shoulder and separated symmetrically. Hands fall naturally.

(1) The upper part of the body bends with right hand over the left knee.

(2) Straighten the upper part of the body and flex both knees into a squat. Raise the left hand in front of the body and keep palm up with eyes looking at the back of hand.(Fig.3-38)

(3) The upper part of the body bends and keep legs straight. Put the left hand over the right knees to reach the right hand.

(4) Return to the commencing position.

(5)-(8) are the same with (1)-(4) but in the opposite direction.

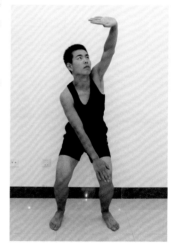

Fig.3-38

【Frequency】

2-4 sets of 8 beats.

【Arrival of qi】

You will feel soreness and swelling in the neck, shoulder, lower back and leg when looking at the back of the hand.

【Application】

It is applicable for soreness, swelling and pain in neck, shoulder, lower back and leg and limb muscle atrophy.

3.1.3.5 Tucking the hand in front of chest

Stand with hands falling relaxed.

(1) Move left foot forward for 1 step and change the center of gravity to left leg. Lift the right heel and raise both arms with palms facing each other. Raise chest and head.

(2) The arms fall along each side of the body while lifting the right knee. Embrace the right knee tightly with both hands with chest. Straighten left leg. (Fig.3-39)

(3) Return to action (1).

(4) Return to the commencing position.

(5)-(8) are the same with (1)-(4) but in the opposite direction.

【Frequency】

2-4 sets of 8 beats.

【Arrival of qi】

You will feel soreness and swelling in the posterior muscles of supporting leg and in the anterior muscles of embraced leg.

3.1.3.6 Roaming at the great pass

Stand upright and put both hands upon the hip with thumbs facing backward.

(1) Move left foot forward for 1 step and land the heel first. Lift right heel and change center of gravity to left leg.(Fig.3-40)

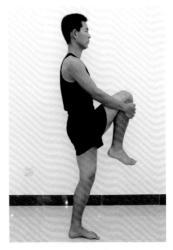

Fig.3-39

(2) Land right heel and flex right knee slightly. Change center of gravity to right leg. Land left heel and bend back of left foot.(Fig.3-41)

(3) Move right foot forward for 1 step. Land the heel and bend back of right foot.

(4) Move center of gravity forward to right leg and lift left heel.

(5) Move center of gravity backward to left leg and bend left knee while lifting right sole.

(6) Straighten left leg and step right leg backward for 1 step. Slightly bend right knee and change center of gravity to right leg.

(7) Return to the commencing position.

【Frequency】

2-4 sets of 8 beats. Start the second set of 8 beats from stepping forward for 1 step of the

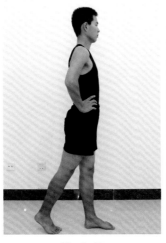

Fig.3-40

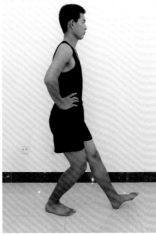

Fig.3-41

right foot.

【Arrival of qi】

You will feel soreness and swelling in left leg and right ankle when the center of gravity lies in left leg; and feel soreness and swelling in right leg and left ankle when the center of gravity lies in right leg.

【Application】

It is applicable for soreness and pain in two legs and difficulty in joint activities.

3.1.4 Exercises for prevention and treatment of the pain on the joints

The training exercises mainly include limb and joint movements, which can smooth the joints, eliminate pain, improve the nervous system function, increase limb muscle strength and maintain the normal body shape.

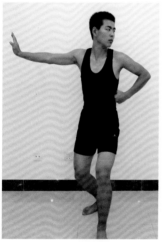

3.1.4.1 Pushing palm in horse stance

Stand upright with legs apart and separated symmetrically, with hands clenching upon hips.

(1) Turn upper part of body to the left posterior direction. Rotate right foot inwards for 45 degree and left foot outwards for 180 degree.

(2) Make a squat into seated stance.(Fig.3-42)

(3) Push right hand to the side of body and push out left elbow to the left while looking at the left.

(4) Return to the commencing position.

(5)-(8) are the same with (1)-(4) but in the opposite direction.

Fig.3-42

【Frequency】

2-4 sets of 8 beats.

【Arrival of qi】

You will feel soreness and swelling in knees, ankles and legs.

3.1.4.2 Dredging up and down

Stand with hands gently clenching upon hip.

(1) Raise right hand with palm up and eyes looking at the back of hand.

(2) Turn body to the left for 90 degree.(Fig.3-43)

(3) The upper part of the body bends with center of right palm to reach outside of left feet passing the hip.(Fig.3-44)

(4) Turn upper part of body to the right and touch the back of 2 feet. Return to the

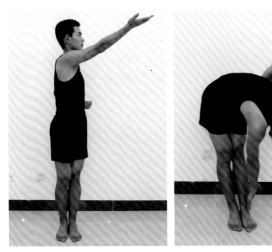

| Fig.3-43 | Fig.3-44 |

commencing position along outside of right leg.

(5)-(8) are the same with (1)-(4) but in the opposite direction.

【Frequency】

2-4 sets of 8 beats.

【Arrival of qi】

You will feel soreness and swelling in the shoulders, back, lower back and legs.

3.1.4.3   Looking back with turn around

Stand upright with legs separated by a big step with hands clenching upon hip.

(1) Turn upper part of body to the left posterior direction. Rotate right foot inwards for 45 degree and left foot outwards for 150 degree.

(2) Flex left knee into a bow stance.(Fig.3-45)

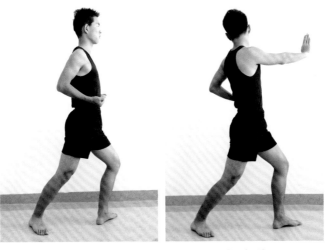

| Fig.3-45 | Fig.3-46 |

(3) Push right arm and palm forward to parallel right leg. Push out left elbow backwards and turn body to the left with head turning to opposite direction.(Fig.3-46)

(4) Return to the commencing position.

(5)-(8) are the same with (1)-(4) but in the opposite direction.

【Frequency】

2-4 sets of 8 beats.

【Arrival of qi】

You will feel soreness and swelling in the neck, shoulders, lower back and legs.

3.1.4.4　Driving legs left and right

Stand upright with legs apart, and put both hands upon the hip with thumbs backward.

(1) Flex left knee and raise the leg. Kick the leg to right anterior direction.(Fig.3-47; Fig.3-48)

(2) Return to the commencing position.

(3) and (4) are the same with (1) and (2) but change to right leg.

【Frequency】

2-4 sets of 8 beats.

【Arrival of qi】

You will feel soreness and swelling in the legs.

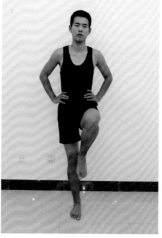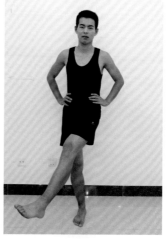

Fig.3-47　　　　　　　　　　　Fig.3-48

3.1.4.5　Kicking shuttlecock all sides

Stand upright and put both hands upon the hip with thumbs backward.

(1) Raise left knee with inner side of foot back kicking upward.(Fig.3-49)

(2) Raise right knee with inner side of foot back kicking upward.

(3) Flex the left knee with outer side of foot back kicking upward.(Fig.3-50)

(4) Flex the right knee with outer side of foot back kicking upward.

(5) Raise left knee and kick forward.(Fig.3-51)

(6) Raise right knee and kick forward.

(7) Flex left knee with heel kicking the hip.(Fig.3-52)

(8) Flex right knee with heel kicking the hip. Return to the commencing position after each action immediately.

【Frequency】

2-4 sets of 8 beats.

【Arrival of qi】

You will feel soreness and swelling in the legs.

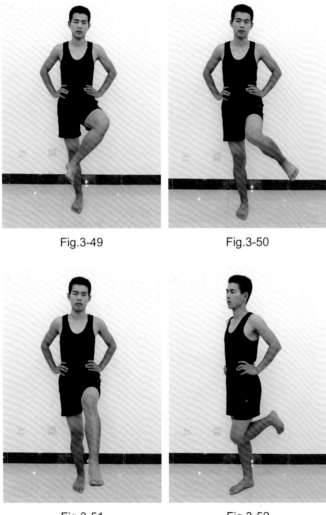

Fig.3-49　　　　　　　　　Fig.3-50

Fig.3-51　　　　　　　　　Fig.3-52

3.1.5 Exercises for prevention and treatment of the tenosynovitis

The training exercises mainly include upper limb movements, which can smooth the shoulder, elbow, wrist and finger joints, improve the blood circulation and nervous control of the soft tissue of upper limbs and have certain functions in prevention and treatment of tennis elbow, wrist and finger tenosynovitis, etc.

3.1.5.1 Pushing palm all sides

Stand upright with legs apart with hands gently clenching upon hips.

(1) Turn both palms and push upward with 4 fingers close together and *Hukou*(the part between thumb and the four fingers) open. Look at the back of hand.(Fig.3-53)

(2) Return to the commencing position.

(3) Push both hands to each side and turn upper part of body to the left with heart of palms to the outside. Look at the back of left hand.(Fig.3-54)

(4) Return to the commencing position.

(5) Is same to (3) but in the opposite direction.

(6) Return to the commencing position.

(7) Push both palms to each side of body with palm up and heart of palm to the outside.

(8) Return to the commencing position.

【Frequency】

2-4 sets of 8 beats.

【Arrival of qi】

You will feel soreness and swelling in the neck, shoulder, elbow, wrist and finger.

3.1.5.2 String stretched back like shooting an arrow

Stand with hands falling relaxed.

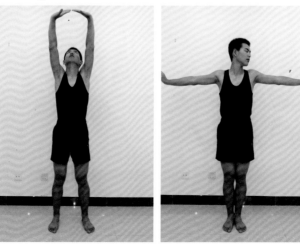

Fig.3-53   Fig.3-54

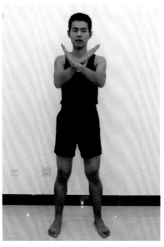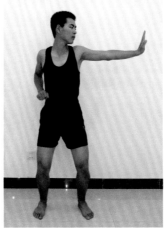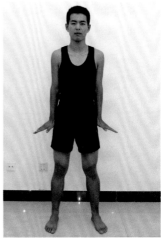

| Fig.3-55 | Fig.3-56 | Fig.3-57 |

(1) Take a step left with left foot and separate 2 feet symmetrically. Cross both palms 30 cm in front of the chest with palm up.(Fig.3-55)

(2) Make a squat and push left hand to the left with palm up and heart of palm to the outside while looking at the back of left hand. Flex right arm and push backward and make a fist with heart of fist downward.(Fig.3-56)

(3) Turn fists into palms and press both palms downward with heart of the palms downward and straighten both legs.(Fig.3-57)

(4) Return to the commencing position.

(5)-(8) are the same with (1)-(4) but in the opposite direction.

【Frequency】

2-4 sets of 8 beats.

【Arrival of qi】

You will feel soreness and swelling in the forearm, wrist and finger.

3.1.5.3　Rotating wrist with arms spread

Stand with hands clenching upon hip. Keep heart of fists upward.

(1) Flex and raise the arms with heart of palms facing each other and head up.

(2) Make fists of both hands and turn heart of fists to outside.(Fig.3-58) Fall both arms along each side of body and return to the commencing position. Perform 1-2 sets of 8 beats first.

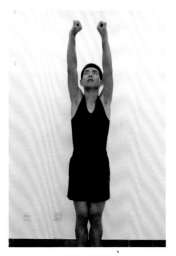

Fig.3-58

(3) Turn both fists to palms and stretch both arms downward with heart of palms facing outside. Raise the arms by each side of body with palms facing each other and head up.

(4) Turn both palms to fists and flex the elbow with the back of fists facing each other. Flex the arms and fall in front of the body and return to the commencing position. Perform another 1-2 sets of 8 beats.

【Frequency】

2-4 sets of 8 beats for each.

【Arrival of qi】

You will feel soreness and swelling in the shoulder, arm, elbow and wrist.

3.1.5.4 Stretching arms forward and backward

Stand upright with legs apart and hands clenching upon hip.

(1) Turn right fist to palm and palm up. Push the palm in the oblique upward direction with heart of palms facing forward and *Hukou*(the part between thumb and the four fingers) open. Turn left fist inward and stretch backward with heart of fist facing upward and look at the heart of fist.(Fig.3-59; Fig.3-60)

(2) Return to the commencing position.

(3) and (4) are the same with (1) and (2) but in the opposite direction.

【Frequency】

2-4 sets of 8 beats.

【Arrival of qi】

You will feel soreness and swelling in the shoulder, arm, elbow, finger and chest.

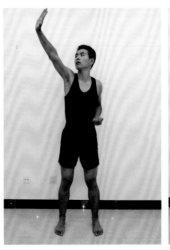 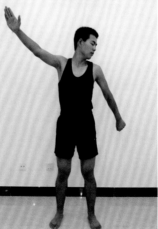

Fig.3-59   Fig.3-60

3.1.5.5 Punching fist in horse stance

Stand upright with legs apart and separated symmetrically with hands clenching upon hips.

(1) Make a squat and push left fist forward with heart of fist facing downward.(Fig.3-61)

(2) Turn left fist into palm and return to the commencing position.

(3) and (4) are the same with (1) and (2) but pushing out right fist.

【Frequency】

2-4 sets of 8 beats.

【Arrival of qi】

You will feel soreness and swelling in the arm, wrist, finger and leg.

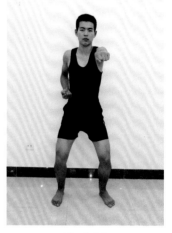

Fig.3-61

3.1.5.6 Rotating waist with relaxed arm

Stand upright with legs apart and both hands fall relaxed.

(1) Raise both arms to form a horizontal line and turn waist to the left.(Fig.3-62)

(2) *Hukou*(the part between thumb and the four fingers) of right hand touches left shoulder with eyes looking at left and attach the back of left hand to waist.(Fig.3-63)

(3) and (4) are the same with (1) and (2) but in the opposite direction.

【Frequency】

2-4 sets of 8 beats.

【Arrival of qi】

You will feel soreness and swelling in the neck, shoulder, elbow, wrist and waist.

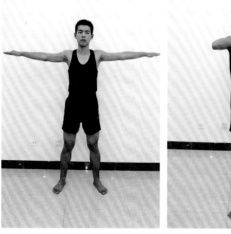
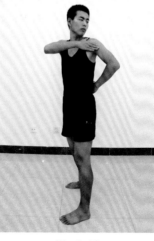

Fig.3-62   Fig.3-63

3.1.6   Exercises for prevention and treatment of the disorder of visceral function

The training exercises mainly include point massage, limb and body movements, which can improve blood circulation, dredge the meridians, improve the neurohumoral regulation function, enhance vitality of the brain and visceral organs and improve metabolism.

3.1.6.1   Rubbing face and kneading grain

Stand upright with legs apart and both hands fall relaxed.

Part one:

(1) Rub from *Dicang*(ST4), to *Yingxiang*(LI20), *Bitong*(EX-HN8), *Jingming*(BL1), *Yintang*(GV29) respectively, until upper eyebrow with the middle fingers of both hands. Separate two hands and rub from *Taiyang*(EX-HN5) downward hardly, circle along the jawbone with thumbs for 1 circle. (Fig.3-64)

(2)-(4) are the same to (1).

(5) Rub the face upwards with 2 palms until hairline and rub from *Baihui*(GV20) to *Fengchi*(GB20). Press root of the 2 palms to the back of ears and then circle along the inner side of jawbone for 1 circle.(Fig.3-65)

(6)-(8) are the same to (5).

【Frequency】

1-2 sets of 8 beats.

Part two:

Press left palm on the upper abdomen tightly and look forward. Touch the palate with tongue and rub the sleep point on the left hand (which lies between the 1st and 2nd metacarpus, in the middle of the line connecting *Hegu*(LI4) and *Sanjian*(LI3), on the

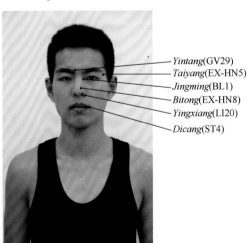

Yintang(GV29)
Taiyang(EX-HN5)
Jingming(BL1)
Bitong(EX-HN8)
Yingxiang(LI20)
Dicang(ST4)

Fig.3-64

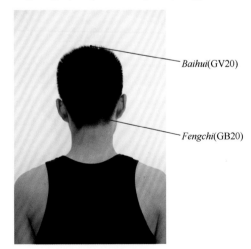

Baihui(GV20)

Fengchi(GB20)

Fig.3-65

large intestine meridian of hand-*yangming* with right thumb for 2-4 times. (Fig.3-66)

【Frequency】

1-2 sets of 8 beats.

【Arrival of qi】

You will feel soreness and swelling locally when rubbing the sleep point and feel hot when rubbing the face.

3.1.6.2　Massage on the chest and abdomen

Stand upright with legs apart and put both hands on upper abdomen with right palm root pressing tightly on the back of left hand.

Rub on the upper abdomen with both hands clockwise for 8 small circles and then rub from upper abdomen, to

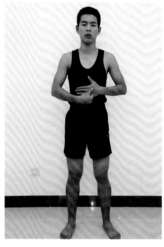

Fig.3-66

hypochondrium, xiphoid process at anterior abdomen until lower abdomen clockwise for 4 big circles. Then perform anticlockwise massage from big to small circles, each for 8 times.(Fig.3-67)

【Arrival of qi】

You will feel warm in the abdomen and unblocked in the chest, sometimes accompanied by belching but feeling more clear and comfortable.

3.1.6.3　Combing hairs with rotating waist

Stand upright with legs apart and both hands falling relaxed.

(1) Attach right palm root to the top of head tightly and comb from hairline, to point *Fengchi*(GB20) with 4 fingers. Flex left elbow and attach back of the hand to waist.(Fig.3-68)

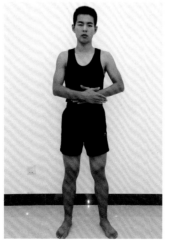
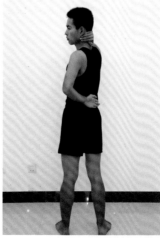

Fig.3-67　　　　　　　　　　　　Fig.3-68

(2) Turn upper part of body to the left and comb *Fengchi*(GB20) with 4 fingers of right hand horizontally for several times.

(3) Rub from *Fengchi*(GB20) forward to *Shuaigu*(GB8) for several times.

(4) Rub from *Fengchi*(GB20) to *Taiyang*(EX-HN5) for several more times and return to the commencing position.

(5)-(8) are the same with (1)-(4) but in the opposite direction.

【Frequency】

2-4 sets of 8 beats.

【Arrival of qi】

You will feel comfortable in the head.

3.1.6.4　Holding palms with knee lifting

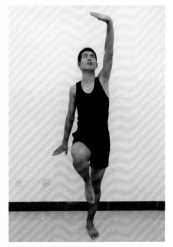

Stand with hands clenching upon lower back.

(1) Move center of gravity to left foot, raise left arm with palm upward, thumb facing inward, *Hukou*(the part between thumb and the four fingers) open and eyes looking at hand back. Meanwhile turn right fist to palm and press downward with fingertips facing forward. Raise right knee and bend the hip.(Fig.3-69)

(2) Return to the commencing position.

(3) and (4) are the same with (1) and (2) but in the opposite direction.

【Frequency】

2-4 sets of 8 beats.

Fig.3-69　　　　【Arrival of qi】

You will feel soreness and swelling in the shoulders, arms and legs.

3.1.6.5　Pitching with rotating waist

Stand upright with legs apart and both hands clenching upon hip.

(1) Turn palms facing downward, turn into fists and raise from each side of body. Look at back of hands and keep *Hukou* (the part between thumb and the four fingers) open and facing each other.(Fig.3-70)

(2) Arms fall a long side of body and put hands over the hip with 2 middle fingers touching each other.

(3) Turn upper part of body to the left and back with eyes looking at the left and back. (Fig.3-71)

(4) Turn upper part of body to the right and back with eyes looking at the right and back.

(5) Return to (2).

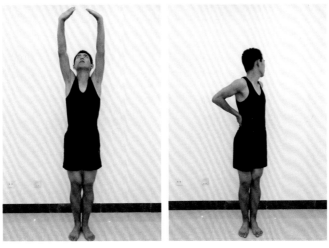

Fig.3-70   Fig.3-71

(6) Make a bow with eyes looking at the ground. (Fig.3-72)

(7) Lean backward with upper part of body with eyes looking upward. (Fig.3-73)

(8) Return to the commencing position.

【Frequency】

1-2 sets of 8 beats.

【Arrival of qi】

You will feel soreness and swelling in the neck, shoulders, lower back and legs.

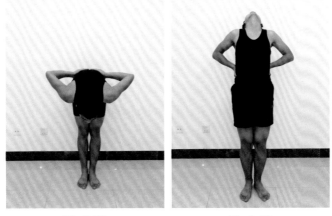

Fig.3-72   Fig.3-73

3.1.6.6   Spreading arms to relax chest

Stand upright with legs apart and both hands falling relaxed.

(1) Raise crossed arms in front of body, lift the heels and inhale with head up. (Fig.3-74)

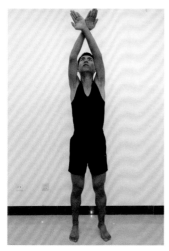

Fig.3-74

(2) Fall the crossed arms in front of body, return to the commencing position, land the heels and exhale.

(3) and (4) are the same with (1) and (2) but in the opposite direction.

【Frequency】

2-4 sets of 8 beats.

【Arrival of qi】

You will feel comfortable in the chest.

【Function and principle】

Prevention and treatment of pain, activity disorders and other diseases in soft tissue of neck, shoulder, low back and leg. These diseases are often caused by wind, cold, wet, strain or trauma. But the common pathology is mainly qi stagnation and blood stasis, resulting in spasm, adhesion, contracture and other pathological phenomena in muscle, fascia, tendon and other soft tissue. The eighteen training exercise stresses "internal strength", requires "obtaining qi with awareness, generate strength with qi and robust the limbs with strength", so as to promote "blood circulation by qi circulation", and change the state of "qi stagnation and blood stasis". Whether there was arrival of qi (that is, acid, swelling, weight and other feelings) locally is a standard to measure if the practitioner has exerted "internal strength".

The arrival of qi during or at the end of the routine shows that the exercise has been successful and the body has benefited.

【Cautions】

Patients can either choose full set or part of the exercise according to the site and severity of lesion.

3.2　Baduanjin Exercise on the bed

Jin(brocade) is weaved with silks of various colors. The ancients regarded the physical exercise actions they created as brocade, as both of them are colorful and pleasing to the eyes. The physical exercise actions is composed of 8 parts, so are called Baduanjin, indicating the action is concise and effective. There are two types of Baduanjin in its long history as Baduanjin in standing position and Baduanjin in sitting position. Here what we introduce belongs to Baduanjin in sitting position, which mainly include massage actions.

3.2.1　General requirements

(1) *Posture*

The Baduanjin Exercise on bad can be carried out sitting on bed, sitting on a chair or lying according to conditions. However, it is best to be naked, or at least be uncovered in the upper part of the body and limbs. If the exercises are carried out from Spring to Winter time, the exercises should be carried out naked for best results. If one lacks exercises or is not healthy enough, or cannot adapt to the cold weather, he or she can do it in the quilt on a bed. These actions the arch of the feet and leg bath are difficult to do, however those who insist on these exercises will have very good results. There is still certain efficacy. Whether sitting or lying to do the exercise depends on the health status, and one should not force himself to accept what he is suitable or not. Otherwise, he will catch cold or other diseases which are bad for the body instead.

When doing the exercise in a lying position, head movements should be done lying on the back with head raised; rubbing arch of the feet should be done sitting with clothes on; rubbing either side of the small of the back should be done lying on the side rubbing with one hand by turns.

(2) *Thought*

It is very important that concentration is placed on the navel while sitting or lying down, thinking nothing but ridding distraction, ears hearing nothing else and eyes looking not far. The navel is located in the middle of the belly which contains viscera and bowels, thus it is effective to concentrate on it.

(3) *Breath*

Take several deep breaths after adjusting posture and thought. Breath refers to the relaxed abdominal breathing, which is comprised of two major types. One is the reverse abdominal breathing, in which the abdomen contracts inward while the chest expands outward during inhalation. The other is called the natural abdominal breathing. The abdomen expands outward and chest contracts inward during inhalation, while the abdomen contracts inward during exhalation. Both being helpful, it would be better to start with the natural abdominal breathing because the reverse type is rather intense. Healthy people may also mix these two breathing methods (use the reserve abdominal breathing before the natural one during every practice, or take natural abdominal breathing this time and reverse abdominal breathing next time).

Inhale through your nose while placing the tongue against palate. Exhale through your mouth when you put down the tongue. Breathe in this way 8 to 9 times (one inhalation and one exhalation are counted as 1 breath, the same method applicable for the followings). Try to make yourself comfortable, relaxed and happy through natural, gentle and smooth breath gradually.

Practice 3 to 5 times at initial tries and then increases the rate as befits you. You can increase 3 times a day to gradually make it to around eighty times every practice if you are willing to do so. But with each increasing in the number of times must be made in view to personal health and in a gradual manner. In particular, caution must be rendered in the case of fragile and sick people. Otherwise, viscera may succumb to injury as a result of the intense ups and downs of diaphragmatic muscle.

Breathing requires fresh indoor air. You may skip deep breathing exercises to practice Baduanjin directly if the indoor air is not fresh (for example, there is not enough time for ventilation in winter). After that, you can get up and dress up, and then take deep breathing in places of fresh air.

After deep breathing, you can practice Baduanjin and Liuduangong Exercise on the bed while always maintain natural breath without intentional efforts.

3.2.2 Basic Movement

Part 1 Dry Bathing

This section is further divided into eight smaller sections for easier mastery. Dry bathing promotes blood circulation, smooths the meridian system, exercises limbs and joints and accelerates gastrointestinal motility. After doing this section, you will feel comfortable and refreshed to great effect.

(1) *Hand bathing*

Clasp your two hands and rub them hot. Grasp the back of the right hand and rub it hard by the left hand, and then grasp the back of the left hand and rub it hard by the right hand. Continue this rubbing movement a dozen times (one left movement and one right movement are counted as one time).(Fig.3-75)

According to the Chinese medicine theory of meridian system, the three yang hand meridians moves from hand to head while the Three Yin Channels of hand moves from the chest to head. Dry bathing should start from hand because it is the enthesis of the three yang meridians of hand and the three yin meridians of hand. By rubbing hands, it helps harmonize qi and blood of hands, makes ten fingers agile and smooths the meridian system in the benefit of further practices.

(2) *Arm bathing*

Press the inner side of the left wrist with the right palm, rub along the arm inner side until the shoulders, and then rub down till to the left hand back along the outer side of the arm. Repeat this movement a dozen times, and rub the right arm by the left hand in the aforesaid method a dozen of times (one back and one forth are counted as one time). (Fig.3-76)

With three important joints, the arm constitutes major collateral channels. Therefore, any discomfort in this part shall have a great bearing on the whole bodies activities. Arm bathing can make joints more flexible, clear and activate the channels and collaterals, and prevent arthritis and arm ache.

People suffering from arm ache resulting from catching cold can practice this exercise. It could be increased to dozens of times, or even hundreds of times to achieve significant effect. However, people, painful from swelling and hot arm due to inflammation should not do so.

(3) *Head bathing*

Rub down to the lower jaw with a little force, and then to the two ears behind the head, gently rub over the head, and back to the forehead. This is one time. Repeat this a dozen times.(Fig.3-77; Fig.3-78)

Then, rub the hair roots of the head with finger pulps or nails of the ten hands evenly and gently 10 to 20 times. And then stroke toward the head with the two thumbs from the vicinity of the temple until to the top before stroking toward the neck, that is, stroking downwards with the closely-drawn five fingers. This is one time.(Fig.3-79; Fig.3-80) Stroking a dozen times helps lower blood pressure. Increase the stroking times by 30 to 70 times if you have a high blood pressure.

Head is where all Yang meets and hundreds of veins pass, therefore needed special care. Head bathing exercise helps promote all Yang rise, harmonize hundreds of veins, and prevent qi and blood aging. Hence, people doing head bathing exercise for a long time are still blessed with rosy complexion when they become old.

Thanks to the connection between hair follicles and blood vessels tips, gently rubbing hair can improve the head peripheral blood circulation, which not only helps prevent

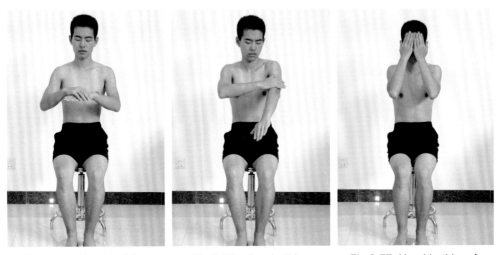

Fig.3-75　Hand bathing　　　Fig.3-76　Arm bathing　　　Fig.3-77　Head bathing Ⅰ

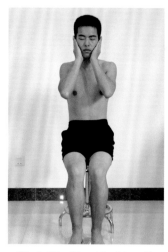

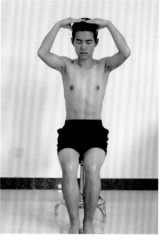

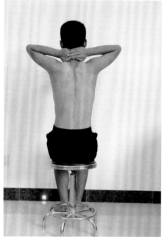

Fig.3-78　Head bathing Ⅱ　　　Fig.3-79　Head bathing Ⅲ　　　Fig.3-80　Head bathing Ⅳ

cerebral hemorrhage, but also overcomes cerebral ischemia through inducing blood up. Stroking your hair frequently may also help hair regrowth because hair rubbing can directly activate its physiological function.

(4) *Eye bathing*

Clench both fists gently, bend two thumbs, and rub the two upper eyelids with the thumb back a dozen times (Fig.3-81). And then spin and rub the two sides of the temple 10 times with the two thumbs, respectively, and rub another 10 times in the reverse direction (Fig.3-82). Finally, pinch the middle of the two eyebrows with the right hand thumb and forefinger and pull a dozen times while stroke from the back-end hairline to the neck with the left hand a dozen times. Repeat the same movement using the other hand a dozen times. (Fig.3-83).

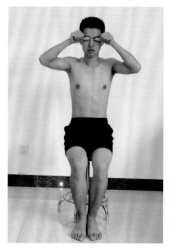

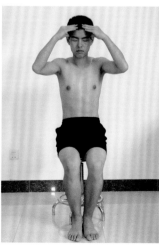

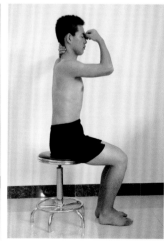

Fig.3-81　Eye bathing Ⅰ　　　Fig.3-82　Eye bathing Ⅱ　　　Fig.3-83　Eye bathing Ⅲ

According to the Chinese medicine theory, the eye's function is related to the five internal organs. Therefore, people suffering from kidney disease often have dim pupils. Eye bathing can smooth eye qi and blood, make muscles remaining plump, and prevent eyelid ptosis. In addition, eye bathing also has some preventive effect on myopia and hyperopia. Because of the plentiful blood capillary around the temple, rubbing this spot can clear and activate the channels and collaterals, and prevent cold invasion. Rubbing makes people feel comfortable, and helps cure headache, dizziness.

Pulling the middle of the two eyes can make deficiency fire inside the eye to remove outside, preventing eye diseases.

(5) *Nose bathing*

Bend thumbs slightly while the other four fingers make a fist. Rub hard 10 times along both sides of the nose bridge with thumbs back and forth (rub up to the eye bottom, and down to the nostril side) (Fig.3-84). Increase the number to over 30 times in winter or during shock chilling weather. While rubbing nose, both hands can rub upward together or downward, or one hand rubs upward while the other downward. One up and one down are counted as one time. Rubbing both sides of the nose could smooth the blood inside the nasal cavity, maintain normal temperature, which makes the intake of air becomes mild, ease the stimulation of cold air in lung so as to prevent colds.

(6) *Breast bathing*

First press the top of the right breast part with the right palm, and push down to the left thigh hard with fingers facing downward. Push hard down to the right thigh from the top of the left breast part with the left hand. Repeat this movement with left hand or right hand, each for a dozen times. (Fig.3-85)

While practicing in the supine position, you can press the right hand at the left breast part

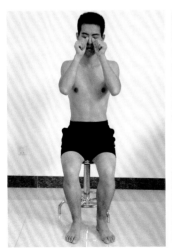 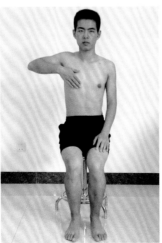 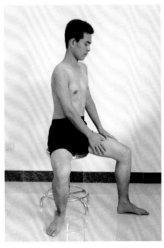

Fig. 3-84　Nose bathing　　Fig.3-85　Breast bathing　　Fig.3-86　Leg bathing

with fingers facing upward, and then rub hard down to the right thigh. Then press the left hand at the right breast part with fingers facing upward and rub hard down to the left thigh. One left and one right are counted as one time. It can rub a dozen times continually.

(7) *Leg bathing*

Grip one side of thigh tight with two hands. Rub hard downward to the ankles and then back to the thigh. Repeat this upward and downward movement a dozen times (one up and one down are counted as one time). The method of rubbing two thighs is the same (Fig.3-86). If there is a feeling any discomfort about this method, you can rub thigh and shank separately.

Leg is the diaphysis bearing the weight of the upper body, and the major roads of the three yang foot meridians and three yin foot meridians. Therefore, leg bathing exercise could make joints flexible, strengthen leg muscle, and helps prevent leg diseases and enhance the ability to walk.

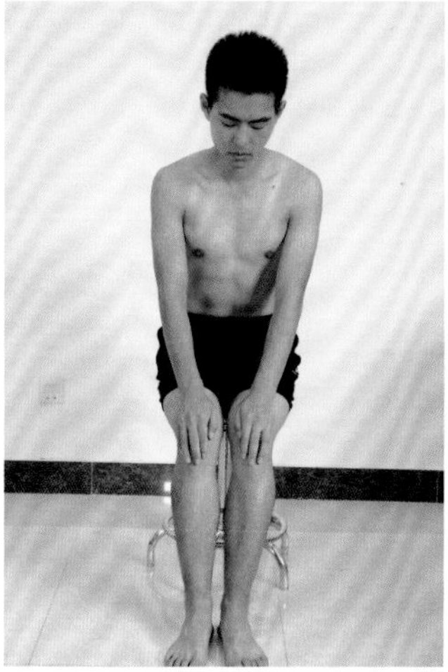

Fig.3-87　Knee bathing

(8) *Knee bathing*

Tightly press the two knees with hand palms, and rotate ten circles outward first and then ten circles inward (Fig.3-87). Knee joints bear the maximum weight during human activities, and have a lot of striated muscles and cartilage ligament tissues but few blood vessels. Therefore, knees hate wetness and coldness, and is prone to strain. Rubbing knees around frequently can increase the knee temperature, expulse coldness, exercise muscles and bones, so as to strengthen knee joints and helps prevent arthritis and other diseases.

Part 2　Occipital-knocking therapy

Press your ear holes firmly with palms and pat your occipital bone gently with the three middle fingers of your hands for a dozen times. Afterwards, put your palms on ear holes gently, press the occipital bone hard and then lift your hands up all of a sudden. Repeat the movement for dozens of times(Fig.3-88). At last, put your middle fingers or index fingers to ear holes, spin 3 times and then pull your fingers out suddenly(Fig.3-89). Repeat the movement for 3 to 5 times.

Since occipital bone represents the place where various yang channels converge and the location of cerebel, gently patting the place can help you keep sober and strengthen your memory. The effect is more obvious especially when you get up early or when you are tired.

In ears, there are nerves like parvis directly linked to the brain, therefore, to plug finger in the ear and pull it out of ear can help the tympanic membrane to vibrate, thus improving listening ability and preventing ear-related diseases.

Part 3　Rolling eyes

Seat still with your head up and back straight. Roll your eyes to the left for 5-6 times and then look straight for a while. Then roll your eyes to the right for 5-6 times and then look straight for a while.

To roll eyes for just a dozen times seems easy and fails to generate marked result. However, it is proofed that as long as you do it in the morning and at the evening for one time respectively, unexpectable result will be achieved after a long time.

Part 4　Clicking teeth

Calm down first and keep focused, and then close your mouth gently and click your upper and lower teeth lightly for three dozen times.

As the end of bones, teeth not only have direct connection with muscles and bones, but are also closely related to the activities of stomach, intestine, spleen, kidney and liver. Therefore, clicking teeth day to day can help to strengthen your teeth and improve the function of the digestive system.

Part 5　Gargling with puffy cheeks

Close your mouth and clench your teeth as if there is something in your mouth, and then move your cheeks and tongue for three dozen times as if you are gargling,which will help to produce much saliva in your mouth. When your mouth is full of saliva, swallow it in three times. At the beginning, perhaps there will have less saliva, but it increases with your practicing time.

Part 6　Rubbing the small of the back

Rub your hands till warm and rub your back hard with your warm hands from the small of the back down to coccygeal end and then to the greatest extend that your legs can reach on your back. Do the same movement for three dozen times. (Fig.3-90)

The small of the back is located within the belt vessel (channels around the waist) and remains the location of kidney, therefore it favors warm and averse cold. Rub your waist with palms will certainly make it warm, which not only keeps the the small of the back warm, but also improves the function of kidney and dredges the belt vessel. If you practice the movement until old, your waist will stand straight and backache can be prevented. People with backache, rub their waist in the way for hundreds of times till sweat and their backache relieved.

Part 7　Kneading abdomen

Abdomen-kneading is useful in case you suffer intestinal problems or chronic intestinal diseases. For men, abdomen-kneading shall be done in the following way: put your left

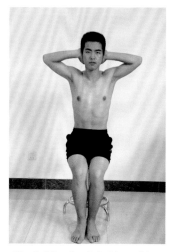 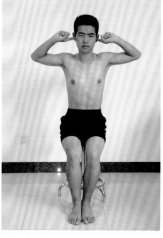 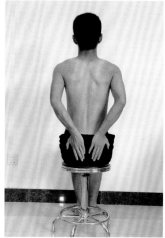

Fig.3-88　Occipital-knocking　　Fig.3-89　Occipital-knocking　　Fig.3-90　Rubbing the small
　　therapy Ⅰ　　　　　　　　　therapy Ⅱ　　　　　　　　　　of the back

hand on your hip or left groin(when you knead your abdomen lying on your back, your hands can place anywhere you like), knead with your right hand from the bottom-left of your xiphoid to your navel, belly and then knead rightward to the starting place. Do it for three dozens of times. Afterwards, put your right hand on your hips or right groin and repeat the above-mentioned movements in opposite direction. Please be gentle while kneading. Since it takes time to knead the abdomen, people without intestinal problems can skip it or just do it for 5 to 6 times. (Fig.3-91)

Though the bowel squirms in a fixed direction, that is downwards, it exists in the cavity of abdomen in a convolution state, which is not fixed in direction, therefore, we need to knead our abdomen for three dozens of times respectively both in the left and right direction. If you keep practicing abdomen-kneading, the digestive function of your intestines and stomach can be improved and diseases related to intestines and stomach can also be prevented. This is because when rubbing stomach and breast, internal organs and diaphragm rise and fall alternately due to outside pressure, which speeds up the movement of intestines and stomach and other organs, thus promoting metabolism, strengthening the function of viscera and bowels and lessening diseases gradually.

Women should practice abdomen-kneading in a different way due to their physical character. For women, one abdomen-kneading goes as follows: rub your palms to warm, put your left hand on your hip (with your thumb located at the back and the other fingers in the front), knead with your right hand from your xiphoid to the bottom-left side and then to the upper side of your navel.You can repeat it for dozens of times (Fig.3-92). Afterwards, put your right hand on your hip, while your left hand from the belly to the bottom-right side through belly (at the edge of pubis) and go back to the belly, which can

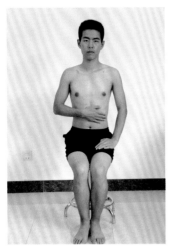
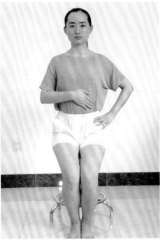
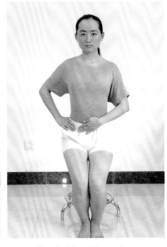

Fig.3-91　Kneading
abdomen Ⅰ

Fig.3-92　Kneading
abdomen Ⅱ

Fig.3-93　Kneading
abdomen Ⅲ

also be repeated for dozens of times(Fig.3-93). The place that the right hand and left hand kneads is different: the right hand kneads between the upper side of the belly and the lower side of xiphoid from the bottom-left side, while the left hand kneads the lower side of belly and belly from the bottom-right side. If women keep practicing the movement,the function of your viscera and bowels will be strengthened, your digestion will be improved and your menstruation will be regulated.

Part 8　Rubbing the arch of the feet

Rub your hands warm and rub the arch of your feet with your hands for more than 80 times(Fig.3-94). There is the kidney meridian of foot-*shaoyin* in the arch of feet. It starts from the arch of feet and stops at the upper chest and it is the position that turbid essence descends. Rubbing the arch of the feet can help to channel the deficiency-type fire in kidney and the turbid essence in the upper body down, soothe the liver and lighten up your eyes. It works better if you rub the arch of the feet after washing your feet.

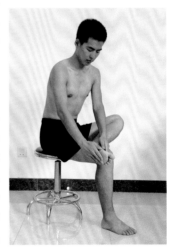

Fig.3-94　Rubbing the
arch of the feet

3.3　The Relaxation Exercise

The Relaxation Exercise is suggested by the former Shanghai Qigong Kurhaus based on the ancients' meditation and mind concentration. It has a focus on mind concentration and guide the Qi with the mind, at the same time combined with slow and soft breathing. Although there is no ancient name, there is a similar cultivation content, such as the concentration and meditation mentioned in the Su Shen Liang Fang, and the relaxation suggested by the modern time Ding Fubao, the progressive relaxation therapy from the US, the relaxation reaction from Japan, and the autosuggestion and relax training from the former Soviet Union. This relaxation is to relax the brain, mind and consciousness by stepped and rhythmical procedures and adjust the body to a natural, relaxed and comfort state, release the tension and exhaustion of the mind and body, reach the balance of tension and relaxation and restore the stamina and vigor. At the same time, it has the effect of gradually concentrating the mind, getting rid of distracting thoughts, relieving uneasiness of the mind, dredging the channels, adjusting the internal organs and help improving the physique and preventing of disease. This relaxation is safe and effective, and not restricted by the surrounding environment, it is easy to learn and practice and it has a quick effect. Suitable for practice when standing, sitting, laying and walking.

The Relaxation Exercise is the basis for getting started with learning Qigong exercises as well as being one of the foundations of entering the state of peace and stable for advanced exercises. This relaxation has a wild range of application and also has better effects on some chronic diseases. Some effect on hypertension, coronary heart disease, glaucoma, asthma, gastrointestinal disease, neurasthenia and other diseases have already been seen, also has the effect of analgesic effect on pain caused by various reasons.

3.3.1   Mind relaxation

Mind relaxation is to make use of the active regulation of the cerebral cortex, with mind and breathing working together, and relax the body from head to feet, or section by section, block by block, or total and partial relaxation. Commonly used methods are:

3.3.1.1   Loosening and mind relaxation

Loosening and mind relaxation is to relax the body from top to bottom, look, listen and think inside the body, at the same time, repeat "loose" and think the part to loosen expand as fermentation and waves so to feel the effect of relaxation.

- Positions: in the standing, seated or lying, or in the walking.
- Breathing: natural or abdominal breathing.
- Mind route: head → neck → shoulder → upper arm → elbow joint → forearm → wrist → hand → chest and back → waist and abdominal → hip joints → thighs → knee → lower legs → ankle → feet.

Think every part, and "loose" 3 times. Then, hands press gently against the abdomen (man: left hand inside; woman: right hand inside) concentrate the mind to the navel and look and listen to it. Concentrate the mind to the point Mingmen between the two kidneys and look and listen to it. Stand still for a moment, wait for the saliva to increase in the mouth and swallow for three times, guide the saliva to the dantian. This is called saliva to the dantian. After that, rub the hands together till hot, and rub your face like washing up and comb your hair, turn your neck slowly, loose your shoulders, move your waist, and take a walk and end.

Operating Tips

Look, listen and think inward when operating, speak silently the word "loose" as moving from part to part and think it loosen like fermentation. Drive the expansion with the force of thinking of "loosening". The key of this exercise is to feel the loosening and expansion. If the feeling of loosening, easing and clearing could be felt, then the relaxation has taken effect.

This method is to achieve the effect of clearing by loosening, loosening is the key to clearing and clearing is the key to curing diseases for it makes it possible for the foul to sank and the clear to rise thus the qi and blood flowing freely and the body becomes agile.

In addition, jade fluid swallowing helps to invigorate stomach, improve digestion, treat indigestion and other illnesses. It also boosts the vital essence, rise the water in kidney, and sank the fire in the heart, once the balance of water and fire is achieved the abdomen will be in the state of excess and the chest and heart will be lightened.

3.3.1.2 Three-route relaxation

Three-route relaxation is to first divide the body into three route: the two sides, the back and the front; each route has 9 part to relax, 4 points to rest, relax them in order when exercising. As one of the basic method of the relaxation exercises, this method is suitable for novice who find it hard to concentrate the mind.

- Position: novices should take supine or seated position for better relaxation effect while adepts could take the position of standing, sitting, laying and walking when exercising.
- Breathing: start with natural breathing and gradually working towards abdominal breathing. Combine breathing and meditation together, think of the part to loosen when inhaling and think of the same part loosening when exhaling, at the same time, think the part to loosen as soft as sponge.
- The mind: the concentration of the mind move as moving to the next point to loosen, guide the qi and loosening with the mind and feel the microscopic alternation after

loosening.

The first route: loosen both sides of the head → both sides of the neck → shoulders → the two upper arms → the two elbow joints → two forearms → hands and concentrate on the point *Zhongchong*(PC1) at the tip of the middle fingers for 1~2 minutes.

The second route: facial loosening → anterior neck loosening → chest loosening → abdomen loosening → two front thigh loosening → both knees → the two lower legs → insteps → big toe loosening, concentrate on the point *Dadun*(LR1) at the tip of the big toe for 1~2 minutes.

The third route: loosening the back head → back of the neck → back → waist loosening → back of the thigh → back of the two lower legs → heel loosening → sole heart loosening. Keep the focus of attention the sole heart and concentrate on the point *Yongquan*(KI1) for 1~2 minutes.

Operating Tips

Breathing, mind and meditation combined closely and feel the loosening. If you are not feeling the loosening, build up tension in all the limbs first and relax suddenly to feel the loosening, this way helps the feeling to appear.

Close the training

Withdraw the mind after finishing all three routes, and concentrate on the dantian point at the navel for 3~5 minutes to close the training.

3.3.1.3　Section by section relaxation

Divide the whole body into several sections and relax from top to bottom, there are usually two ways of sectioning.

- The head → shoulders, arms and hands → chest → abdomen → legs → feet.
- The head → neck → two upper limbs → abdomen, chest, back and waist → both thighs → lower legs and feet.

Focus the attention on one section and meditate "loose" twice to three times, move to the next section and cycle back twice to three times and stop at the navel. This method is for novices who find it hard to memorize the many points of the routes.

3.3.1.4　Partial relaxation

This method is based on the three-route relaxation, focus on a specific affected point or point of tension and meditate "loose" for 20 to 30 times. This method is for those have already mastered the three-route relaxation and have an affected part of tension point to loosen, for example, the eyes of glaucoma patients or livers of the hepatopathy patients.

3.3.1.5 Overall relaxation

Think the whole body as one part and relax. There are 3 methods in overall relaxation.

- Like falling water, relax from top to feet.
- Take navel as the center of the body, relax forth outward and repeat "loose".
- Follow the routes of the three-route relaxation and relax down each route without stop.

This method is suitable for those capable of adjusting the body, emotionally stable and mastered the three-route relaxation and section by section relaxation. Or novice who have problem with the three-route relaxation and section by section relaxation. Or patients with too much Yang in liver, too less Yin and too much fire or too much topside and too little downside.

3.3.1.6 Reversing relaxation

Relax the body in to reverse route.

The first route: sole → heel → back of the lower legs → popliteal fossa → thigh back → tail bone → waist → back → back of the neck → back of the head → top of the head.

The second route: sole → instep → front of the lower legs → knees → front thigh → abdomen → chest → front of the neck → face → top of the head.

3.3.2 Vibrating relaxation

In a natural standing position, breath evenly and think the body as a bird net and shake the foul down under the ground. Shake and vibrate the whole body for 2 to 5 minutes at the frequency of 130 to 160 times per minutes, focus on the wrists, ankles and heels. After that stand still for 3 to 6 minutes, extend the period of still standing according to the patient's condition or exercise other methods.

Clinical practice has shown that rhythmical vibration has the effect of sinking, adjusting and lowering Qi. This exercise associates activity and inertia, practice this method with persevere not only helps to keep fit but also have salience effects on hyperactivity of liver-*yang* and excess in the upper and deficiency in the lower diseases like hypertension, vascular headache, menopause, neurasthenia syndrome, etc. Vibration is often used as preparations and guiding method for other exercises. Vibrating the hands and feet helps to regulate the 12 channels and integral organs. Those not suitable for other exercises can reach the state of peace and relaxation with this method.

3.3.3 Tapping relaxation

This manipulation is for Qigong novices or those can't get relaxed by other manipulations, by tapping, which mobilizes inner movements with outer movements, some effects are easy to emerge. The effects would be better if combine tapping relaxation with points pressing manipulation. Tap from head to feet, section by section and with rhythm, repeat "relax" to guide towards relaxation.

Tapping route: Head → neck → shoulders → elbow joints → back of hands → fingers → chest and abdominal → back and waist → hips → both thighs → knees → insteps → toes.

〖Appendix〗

Meridians and Points Query Table

Name of the meridians	Name of the points	Location	Indications
The Lung Meridian of Hand-Taiyin	Zhongfu(LU1)	6 *cun* lateral to the anterior midline and at the same level of the first intercostal space.	①Cough, asthma, fullness in the chest; ②Chest pain and upper back pain.
	Yunmen(LU2)	On the upper lateral chest, superior to the Processus coracoideus, in the depression of the infraclavicular fossa, 6 *cun* lateral to the anterior midline .	①Cough, asthma, chest pain; ②Shoulder and upper back pain.
	Tianfu(LU3)	On the radial border of the biceps muscle, 3 *cun* below the front end of the axillary fold.	①Cough, asthma, nosebleed; ②Goiter; ③Pain in the upper arm.
	Xiabai(LU4)	On the radial side of the tendon of the biceps muscle, 4 *cun* below the front end of the axillary fold.	①Cough, asthma, nausea; ②Pain in the upper arm.
	Chize(LU5)	On the transverse crease of the elbow, in the radial depression of the tendon of the biceps muscle.	①Cough, asthma, fullness in the chest, coughing up blood, nosebleed, sore throat, fever, infantile convulsion, acute vomiting and diarrhea; ②Pain in the elbow and arm.
	Kongzui(LU6)	On the medial side of the forearm, along the line linking *Taiyuan*(LU9) and *Chize*(LU5), 7 *cun* above the transverse crease of the wrist.	Cough, coughing up blood, asthma, nosebleed, sore throat, hemorrhoids, spasm and pain in the arm.
	Lieque(LU7)	On the upper edge of the styloid process of the radius, 1.5 *cun* above the transverse crease of the wrist.	Cough, asthma, rigidity of nape with headache, deviation mouth and eyes, sore throat, toothache, pain in the wrist.
	Jingqu(LU8)	In the depression between the styloid process of the radius and the radial side, 1 *cun* above the transverse crease of the wrist.	①Cough, asthma, chest pain; ②Swelling and pain in the throat; ③Pain in the wrist.
	Taiyuan(LU9)	On the radial side of the transverse crease of the wrist, in the depression of the lateral side of the radial artery.	Cough, asthma, coughing blood, chest pain, sore throat, acrotism, pain in the wrist.
	Yuji(LU10)	On the midpoint of the 1st metacarpal bone, dorso-vental boundary of hand.	Cough, coughing up blood, sore throat, sudden aphonia, fever.
	Shaoshang (LU11)	On the radial side of the thumb, about 0.1 *cun* from the corner of the fingernail.	Sore throat, nosebleed, high fever, unconsciousness, cough.

Name of the meridians	Name of the points	Location	Indications
The Pericardium Meridian of Hand-Jueyin	Tianchi(PC1)	On the chest, in the 4th intercostal space, 1 *cun* lateral to the nipple, 5 *cun* lateral to the anterior midline.	① Mastitis, insufficient lactation; ② Cough, asthma; ③ Pain in the chest and heart.
	Tianquan(PC2)	On the palmar side of the upper arm，2 *cun* below the level of the anterior axillary fold, between the two heads of the biceps brachii muscle.	① Cardiodynia, cough, distention in the chest; ② Pain in the chest, upper back, and medial side of the upper arm.
	Quze(PC3)	On the transverse cubital crease, on the ulnar side of the tendon of the biceps muscle of the arm.	Cardiodynia, palpitations, stomachache, vomiting, sunstroke, pain in the elbow and arm.
	Ximen(PC4)	On the palmar side of the forearm, 5 *cun* above the transverse crease of the wrist, and between the tendons of the palmaris longus and flexor carpi radialis.	Cardiodynia, palpitations, restlessness, chest pain, hemoptysis, hematemesis, epistaxis, furunculosis, epilepsy.
	Jianshi(PC5)	On the palmar side of the forearm, 3 *cun* above the transverse crease of the wrist, and between the tendons of the palmaris longus and flexor carpi radialis.	Cardiodynia, palpitations, stomachache, vomiting, febrile disease, malaria, psychosis, epilepsy.
	Neiguan(PC6)	On the palmar side of the forearm, 2 *cun* above the transverse crease of the wrist, and between the tendons of the palmaris longus and flexor carpi radialis.	Cardiodynia, palpitations, chest pain, oppression in the chest, stomachache, vomiting, stroke, insomnia, dizziness, depression, epilepsy, migraine, febrile disease, pain in the elbow and arm.
	Daling(PC7)	In the middle of the transverse crease of the wrist, and between the tendons of the palmaris longus and flexor carpi radialis.	Cardiodynia, palpitations, stomachache, vomiting, hypochondriac pain, epilepsy, pain in the elbow and arm.
	Laogong(PC8)	In the middle of the palm, between the 2nd and 3rd metacarpal bones.	Stroke and coma, sunstroke, cardiodynia, restlessness, epilepsy, stomatitis, foul breath, tinea manus.
	Zhongchong (PC9)	In the center of the tip of the middle finger.	Stroke and coma, sunstroke, syncope, stiff tongue impeding speech, infantile convulsions, febrile disease.
The Heart Meridian of Hand-Shaoyin	Jiquan(HT1)	At the apex of the axilla, on the pulsation point of the axillary artery.	Palpitations, cardiac pain, fullness in the chest, hypochondriac and costal pain; pain in the shoulder and arm, loss of the use of the upper limb, scrofula.
	Qingling(HT2)	On the medial side of the arm and on the line connecting Jiquan(HT1) and Shaohai(HT3), 3 *cun* above the cubital crease, in the groove medial to the biceps muscle of the arm.	Headache, chill, yellowish eyeballs, hypochondriac pain, pain in the shoulder and arm.

Name of the meridians	Name of the points	Location	Indications
The Heart Meridian of Hand-Shaoyin	Shaohai(HT3)	With the elbow flexed, in the center between the medial end of the transverse cubital crease and the medial epicondyle of the humerus.	Cardiac pain, hypochondriac pain, pain of the arm and elbow, paralysis of the upper limbs, scrofula.
	Lingdao(HT4)	With the elbow flexed, in the center between the medial end of the transverse cubital crease and the medial epicondyle of the humerus.	① Cardiac pain; ② Axillary and hypochondriac pain; ③ Pain of the arm and elbow, paralysis of the upper limbs; ④ Scrofula.
	Tongli(HT5)	On the palmar aspect of the forearm, 1 *cun* above the *Shenmen*(HT7) point.	Sudden aphonia, aphasia with stiff tongue, palpitations, pain in the wrist and arm.
	Yinxi(HT6)	On the palmar aspect of the forearm, 0.5 *cun* above the *Shenmen*(HT7) point.	Cardiac pain, palpitations, hematemesis, night sweats, aphasia.
	Shenmen(HT7)	On the palmar ulnar end of the transverse crease of the wrist, in the depression on the radial side of the tendon of the flexor carpi ulnaris.	Insomnia, forgetfulness, dementia, psychosis, epilepsy, palpitations, upset, cardiac pain.
	Shaofu(HT8)	On the palm, between the 4th and 5th metacarpal bones, where the tip of the little finger rests when a fist is made.	① Palpitations, chest pain; ② Itching and pain of the genitals; ③ Spasmodic pain of the little finger, heat sensations in the palm.
	Shaochong (HT9)	On the radial side of the little finger, approximately 0.1 *cun* from the corner of the nail.	① Cardiac pain, palpitations; ② Psychosis, coma; ③ Febrile diseases.
The Large Intestine Meridian of Hand-Yangming	Shangyang (LI1)	0.1 *cun* lateral to the radial nail corner of the index ringe.	Toothache, sore throat, coma, sunstroke, febrile disease.
	Erjian(LI2)	In the depression of the radial side, distal to the 2nd metacarpophalangeal joint when a loose fiat is made.	Nosebleed, toothache, red and swollen eyes, deviated mouth and eye, febrile disease.
	Sanjian(LI3)	In the depression of the radial side and proximal to the 2nd metacarpophalangeal joint.	Toothache, nosebleed, sore throat, fever.
	Hegu(LI4)	Between the 1st and 2nd metacarpal bones, approximately in the middle of the 2nd metacarpal bone on the radial side.	Headache, toothache, nosebleed, red and swollen eyes, deafness, deviated mouth and eye, fever and aversion to cold, with or without sweating, amenorrhea, delayed labour, urticaria, paralysis of the forearm, unable to move voluntarily, painful wrist and forearm.
	Yangxi(LI5)	On the transverse crease of the radial side of the wrist, between the tendons of the extensor pollicis longus and brevis.	Headache, toothache, sore throat, pain in the wrist.

Name of the meridians	Name of the points	Location	Indications
The Large Intestine Meridian of Hand-Yangming	*Pianli*(LI6)	With the elbow slightly flexed, on the radial side of the dorsal surface of the forearm and on the line connecting *Yangxi*(LI5) and *Quchi*(LI11), 3 *cun* above the crease of the wrist.	Nosebleed, tinnitus, pain in the forearm, abdominal distending pain, edema.
	Wenliu(LI7)	With the elbow flexed, on the line linking the *Yangxi*(LI5) and *Quchi*(LI11) points, 5 *cun* above the wrist crease.	①Headache, swollen of the face, sore throat; ②Aching shoulders and back; ③Abdominal pain, borborygmus.
	Xialian(LI8)	On the line connecting *Yangxi*(LI5) and *Quchi*(LI11), 4 *cun* below the cubital crease.	Headache, vertigo and pain in the elbow, abdominal distention, abdominal pain, pain in the elbow.
	Shanglian(LI9)	On the line connecting *Yangxi*(LI5) and *Quchi*(LI11), 3 *cun* below the cubital crease .	Pain and numbness in the elbow and arm, paralysis of the forearm, headache, borborygmus, abdominal pain.
	Shousanli (LI10)	On the line linking the *Yangxi*(LI5) and *Quchi*(LI11) points, 2 *cun* below *Quchi*(LI11).	Abdominal pain, diarrhea, toothache, swollen cheek, paralysis of the forearm, pain of the elbow and arm.
	Quchi(LI11)	At the lateral end of the cubital crease with the elbow flexed.	Febrile disease, rubella, eczema, sore throat, toothache, redness and pain in the eyes, abdominal pain, diarrhea, paralysis of the arm, pain and weakness in the elbow.
	Zhouliao(LI12)	With the elbow flexed, 1 *cun* above the *Quchi*(LI11) point, on the border of the humerus.	Aching, numbness and spasm of the elbow and arm.
	Shouwuli (LI13)	On the line connecting *Quchi*(LI11) and *Jianyu*(LI15), 3 *cun* above *Quchi*(LI11).	Spasm and pain of the elbow and arm, scrofula.
	Binao(LI14)	On the lateral side of the arm, at the insertion of the deltoid muscle and 7 *cun* above *Quchi*(LI11).	Painful arm and shoulder, impaired arm movement, eye diseases, scrofula.
	Jianyu(LI15)	With the arm abducted, at the upper border of the deltoid muscle, in the inferior anterior depression of the shoulder.	Pain in the shoulder and arm, impaired movement of arm, rashes.
	Jugu(LI16)	In the upper portion of the shoulder, in the depression between the acromial extremity of the clavicle and the scapular spine.	①Pain of the shoulder and upper back; ②Scrofula, goiter.
	Tianding(LI17)	On the lateral side of the neck, on the posterior border of m.sternocleidomastoideus, at the midpoint of the line linking the *Futu*(LI18) and *Quepen*(ST12) points.	Sore throat, sudden loss of voice, scrofula, goiter.

Name of the meridians	Name of the points	Location	Indications
The Large Intestine Meridian of Hand-Yangming	*Futu*(LI18)	3 *cun* lateral to the tip of the Adam's apple, between the sternal head and clavicular head of m.sternocleidomastoideus.	① Sore throat, sudden loss of voice; ② Scrofula, goiter; ③ Cough and asthma.
	Kouheliao (LI19)	On the upper lip, directly below the lateral border of the nostril, on the level of *Shuigou*(DU26).	Nosebleed, nasal obstruction, deviated face, trismus.
	Yingxiang (LI20)	0.5 *cun* beside the lateral border of the nasal ala, in the nasolabial groove.	Nasal obstruction, facial paralysis, nosebleed, facial itchiness, ascariasis of the biliary tract.
The San Jiao Meridian of Hand-Shaoyang	*Guanchong* (SJ1)	On the ulnar side of the distal segment of the 4th finger, 0.1 *cun* from the corner of the nail.	Headache, red eyes, deafness, sore throat, febrile diseases, coma.
	Yemen(SJ2)	On the dorsum of the hand, proximal to the margin of the web between the 4th and 5th fingers, at the junction of the red and white skin.	Headache, red eyes, tinnitus, deafness, malaria, pain in the upper limbs.
	Zhongzhü (SJ3)	On the dorsum of the hand proximal to the 4th metacarpophalangeal joint, in the depression between the 4th and 5th metacarpal bones.	Headache, red eyes, tinnitus, deafness, sore throat, febrile diseases.
	Yangchi(SJ4)	At the midpoint of the dorsal crease of the wrist, in the depression on the ulnar side of the tendon of the extensor muscle of the finger.	Red and swollen eyes, deafness, sore throat, malaria, diabetes, febrile diseases.
	Waiguan(SJ5)	On the dorsal side of the forearm and on the line connecting *Yangchi* (SJ4) and the tip of the olecranon, 2 *cun* proximal to the dorsal crease of the wrist, between the radius and ulna.	Febrile disease, headache, cheek pain, red and swollen eyes, tinnitus, deafness, scrofula, hypochondriac pain, pain in upper limbs.
	Zhigou(SJ6)	1 *cun* above *Waiguan*(SJ5).	Tinnitus, deafness, sudden loss of voice, scrofula, hypochondriac pain, constipation, febrile disease.
	Huizong(SJ7)	On the dorsal aspect of the forearm, 3 *cun* above the transverse crease of the dorsum of the wrist, on the ulnar side of *Zhigou*(TE6), and on the radial side of the ulna.	① Tinnitus, deafness; ② Epliepsy.
	Sanyangluo (SJ8)	On the dorsal aspect of the forearm, 4 *cun* above the transverse crease of dorsum of the wrist, between the ulna and radius.	① Deafness, sudden loss of voice, toothache; ② Atrophy or paralysis in the upper limbs.
	Sidu(SJ9)	On the dorsal aspect of the forearm, on the line connecting *Yangchi*(SJ4) and tip of the elbow, 5 *cun* below the tip of the elbow between the ulna and radius.	① Numbness and pain of the upper limbs; ② Deafness, sudden loss of voice, toothache, headache.

Name of the meridians	Name of the points	Location	Indications
The San Jiao Meridian of Hand- Shaoyang	Tianjing(SJ10)	On the lateral aspect of the arm, when the elbow is bent, the point is in the depression about 1 *cun* above the olecranon of the ulna.	①Migraine, deafness, epliepsy; ②Scrofula; ③Pain in the elbow and arm.
	Qinglengyuan (SJ11)	On the lateral aspect of the arm, when the elbow is bent, the point is 2 *cun* directly above the tip of the elbow, 1 *cun* above *Tianjing*(SJ10).	①Pain in the shoulder and arm, paralysis of the upper limb; ②Headache, eye pain.
	Xiaoluo(SJ12)	On the lateral aspect of the arm, on the midpoint of the line connecting *Qinglengyuan*(SJ11) and *Naohui*(SJ13).	①Numbness and pain of the upper limbs; ②Headache, toothache, stiff neck; ③Epilepsy.
	Naohui(SJ13)	On the lateral aspect of the arm, on the line connecting the olecranon and *Jianliao*(SJ14), 3 *cun* below *Jianliao*(SJ14), on the posterior and inferior border of the deltoideus.	①Scrofula, goiter; ②Spasm and pain in the upper limbs.
	Jianliao(SJ14)	On the shoulder, posterior to *Jianyu* (LI15), when the arm abducted, in the depression posterior and interior to the acromion.	①Pain in the shoulder and arm, heaviness of the shoulder with inability to raise the arm; ②Pain in the hypochondriac region.
	Tianliao(SJ15)	In the region of the scapula, midway between *Jianjing*(GB21) and *Quyuan*(SI13), on the superior angle of the scapula.	①Pain in the shoulder and arm; ②Spasm of the nape of the neck.
	Tianyou(SJ16)	On the side of the neck, directly inferior to the posterior aspect of the mastoid process, at the level of the angle of the mandible, on the posterior border of the sternocleidomastoideus.	①Headache, stiff neck, dizziness, eye pain, deafness; ②Scrofula.
	Yifeng(SJ17)	Posterior to the ear lobe, in the depression between the mastoid process and the angle of the mandible.	①Tinnitus, deafness; ②Deviation of the mouth and eye, locked jaw, toothache; ③Scrofula.
	Chimai(SJ18)	On the head, posterior to the ear in the center of the mastoid process, at the junction of the middle and lower third of the curved line along the ear helix connecting *Jiaosun*(SJ20) and *Yifeng*(SJ17).	①Migraine, tinnitus, deafness; ②Infantile convulsions.
	Luxi(SJ19)	On the head, at the junction of the upper and middle third of the curved line along the ear helix connecting *Jiaosun*(SJ20) and *Yifeng*(SJ17).	①Migraine, tinnitus, deafness; ②Infantile convulsions.
	Jiaosun(SJ20)	On the head, on the hairline directly above the ear apex where the ear is folded forward.	①Migraine, stiff neck; ②Mumps, cataracts, toothache.

Name of the meridians	Name of the points	Location	Indications
The San Jiao Meridian of Hand- Shaoyang	*Ermen*(SJ21)	Location in front of the supratragic notch, in the depression of the posterior border of the condylar process of the mandible when the mouth is open.	① Tinnitus, deafness; ② Toothache.
	Erheliao(SJ22)	On the side of the head, on the posterior border of the hairline of the temple, at the level with the root of the ear, posterior to the superficial temporal artery.	① Migraine, tinnitus; ② Locked jaw.
	Sizhukong (SJ23)	In the depression of the lateral end of the eyebrow.	① Redness, swelling and pain of the eyes, twitching of the eyelids; ② Migraine; ③ Psychosis and epilepsy.
The Small Intestine Meridian of Hand-Taiyang	*Shaoze*(SI1)	On the ulnar side of the little finger, approximately 0.1 *cun* from the comer of the nail.	Febrile disease, coma, headache, nebula, sore throat, mastitis, agalactia.
	Qiangu(SI2)	At the junction of the red and white skin along the ulnar border of the hand, at the ulnar end of the crease of the 5th metacarpophalangeal joint when a loose fist is made.	Headache, ophthalmalgia, tinnitus, sore throat, febrile disease, acute mastitis.
	Houxi(SI3)	On the ulnar side of the hand, when a loose fist is made, proximal to the 5th metacarpophalangeal joint, at the top of the transverse crease and the junction of the red and white skin.	Stiff nape with headache, lower back pain, red eyes, deafness, sore throat, night sweats, malaria, psychosis, epilepsy.
	Wangu(SI4)	On the ulnar side of the palm, in the depression between the 5th metacarpal bone and the hamate bone, at the junction of the red and white skin.	Rigid nape with headache, tinnitus, deaf, nebula, diabetes, febrile diseases, malaria, pain and spasm in the fingers and wrists.
	Yanggu(SI5)	On the ulnar border of the wrist, in the depression between the styloid process of the ulnar and triangular bone.	Headache, dizziness, tinnitus, deafness, pain in the wrist, febrile diseases, psychosis, epilepsy.
	Yanglao(SI6)	On the dorsal ulnar aspect of the forearm, in the depression on the radial side of the proximal end of the capitulum of the ulna.	① Blurred vision; ② Numbness and pain in the shoulder, back, elbow and arm, stiff neck, acute lumbar pain.
	Zhizheng(SI7)	On the dorsal ulnar aspect of the forearm, 5 *cun* above the dorsal crease of the wrist.	Rigid nape with headache, and fingers, febrile diseases, psychosis, pain in the elbow and forearm.
	Xiaohai(SI8)	With the elbow flexed, in the depression between the olecranon of the ulna and the medial epicondyle of the humerus.	Pain in the elbow and arm, epilepsy, tinnitus, deafness.

Name of the meridians	Name of the points	Location	Indications
The Small Intestine Meridian of Hand-Taiyang	Jianzhen(SI9)	Posterior and inferior to the shoulder joint, 1 *cun* above the posterior end of the axillary fold with the arm abducted.	Numbness and pain in the shoulder and arm,scrofula.
	Naoshu(SI10)	On the shoulder, directly above the posterior end of the axillary fold, in the depression inferior to the scapular spine.	①Pain in the shoulder and arm; ②Scrofula.
	Tianzong(SI11)	In the depression of the center of the subscapular fossa, level with the 4th thoracic vertebra.	Scapular pain, asthma; mastitis.
	Bingfeng(SI12)	In the region of the scapula, in the center of the suprascapular fossa, directly above *Tianzong*(SI11), in the depression when the arm is lifted.	Scapular pain and aching numbness of the upper arm.
	Quyuan(SI13)	In the region of the scapula, on the medial end of the suprascapular fossa, midpoint of the line between *Naoshu*(SI10)and the spinous process of the 2nd thoracic vertebra.	Pain in the scapula, back and neck.
	Jianwaishu (SI14)	3 *cun* lateral to the lower border of the spinous process of the 1st thoracic vertebrae.	Stiffness of nape and back, pain in the shoulder and back.
	Jianzhongshu (SI15)	on the back, 2 *cun* lateral to the lower border of the spinous process of the 7th cervical vertebra.	①Cough, asthma; ②Pain in the shoulder and upper back.
	Tianchuang (SI16)	On the lateral aspect of the neck, on the posterior border of the sternocleidomastoideus, posterior to *Futu*(LI8), and level with the Adam's Apple.	①Sore and swollen throat, sudden loss of voice, tinnitus, deafness; ②Pain and stiffness in the nape of the neck.
	Tianrong(SI17)	Posterior to the mandibular angle in the depression of the anterior border of the sternocleidomastoid muscle.	Tinnitus,deafness,sore and swollen throat, pain and distension in the nape of the neck.
	Quanliao(SI18)	On the face, directly below the outer canthus, in the depression below the zygomatic bone.	Facial paralysis, trembling eyelids, toothache, swollen lips.
	Tinggong (SI19)	On the face, anterior to the tragus and posterior to the mandibular condyloid process, in the depression found when the mouth is open.	Tinnitus, deafness, toothache, epilepsy.
The Spleen Meridian of Foot-Taiyin	Yinbai(SP1)	On the medial side of the great toe and about 0.1 *cun* lateral to the corner of the toenail.	Abdominal distention, diarrhea, blood in the stool, blood in the urine, epilepsy, irritability and mania, profuse dreaming, convulsions, coma, pain in the chest.

continued

Name of the meridians	Name of the points	Location	Indications
The Spleen Meridian of Foot-Taiyin	Dadu(SP2)	In the depression anterior and inferior to the 1st metatarsophalangeal joint of the big toe,at the junction of the red and the white skin.	Abdominal distension, stomach pain, diarrhea, constipation, febrile disease with absence of sweating.
	Taibai(SP3)	On the posterior border of the small head of the 1st metatarsal bone, at the junction of the red and white skin.	Abdominal distention, stomachache, vomiting, constipation, borborygmus, diarrhea, dysentery, heaviness of the body, pain in joints.
	Gongsun(SP4)	On the medial border of the foot, anterior to the proximal end of the first metatarsal, at the junction of the red and white skin.	Stomachache, abdominal pain, vomiting, borborygmus, diarrhea, dysentery, edema, restlessness, insomnia, irritability, somnolence, beriberi.
	Shangqiu(SP5)	In the depression anterior and inferior to the medial malleolus, at the midpoint of the line connecting the tuberosity of the navicular bone and the tip of the medial malleolus.	Abdominal distension, borborygmus, diarrhea, constipation, jaundice, pain in the foot and ankle.
	Sanyinjiao (SP6)	3 cun above the tip of the medial malleolus and on the posterior border of the medial aspect of the tibia.	Irregular menstruation, metrorrhagia, leukorrhea , dysmenorrhea, prolapse of the uterus, sterility, difficult labor, seminal emission, impotence, enuresis, frequent urination, dysuria, abdominal distention, borborygmus, diarrhea, palpitation, insomnia, hypertension, eczema, urticaria,weakness and flaccidity of the lower limbs, yin deficiency.
	Lougu(SP7)	On the line connecting the tip of the medial malleolus and Yinlingquan(SP9),6 cun above the tip of the medial malleolus.	Abdominal distension, borborygmus, seminal emission, weakness and flaccidity of the lower limbs.
	Diji(SP8)	On the line connecting the tip of the medial malleolus and, 3 cun below Yinlingquan(SP9).	Abdominal distension,abdominal pain,diarrhea, dysmenorrhea, uterine bleeding, irregular menstruation,difficulty in micturition, edema.
	Yinlingquan (SP9)	In the depression inferior to the medial condyle of the tibia.	Abdominal distension and pain, diarrhea, difficulty in urination, aconuresis, edema, jaundice, pain in the knees.
	Xuehai(SP10)	When the knee is flexed, 2 cun above the superior medial corner of the patella and on the prominence of the medial head of the quadriceps muscle.	Irregular menstruation, metrorrhagia, dysmenorrhea, amenorrhea, itching of skin, eczema ,urticaria, pruritus, pain in the medial side of the knee and thigh.

Name of the meridians	Name of the points	Location	Indications
The Spleen Meridian of Foot-Taiyin	Jimen(SP11)	On the line connecting Xuehai (SP10)and Chongmen(SP12), 6 cun above Xuehai(SP10).	Dysuria, enuresis, swelling and pain of the groin.
	Chongmen (SP12)	On the lateral end of the inguinal groove, 3.5 cun lateral to the midpoint of the upper margin of the pubic symphysis, on the lateral side of the femoral artery.	①Abdominal pain, hernia; ②Uterine bleeding, leukorrhea.
	Fushe(SP13)	0.7 cun superior and lateral to Chongmen(SP12), 4 cun lateral to the midline of the abdomen.	Abdominal pain, hernia, distension, and masses in the abdomen.
	Fujie(SP14)	1.3 cun below Daheng(SP15), 4 cun lateral to the midline of the abdomen .	Abdominal pain, diarrhea, and constipation.
	Daheng(SP15)	4 cun lateral to the center of the umbilicus.	Abdominal pain, diarrhea, and constipation.
	Fuai(SP16)	3 cun above the center of the umbilicus, 4 cun lateral to the anterior midline of the abdomen .	Abdominal pain, diarrhea, dysentery, constipation, and dyspepsia.
	Shidou(SP17)	In the 5th intercostal space, 6 cun lateral to the anterior midline of the chest.	①Belching, abdominal distension; ②Edema; ③Distension and pain in the chest and hypochondrium.
	Tianxi(SP18)	In the 4th intercostal space, 6 cun lateral to the anterior midline of the chest.	①Chest pain, cough; ②Acute mastitis, insufficient lactation.
	Xiongxiang (SP19)	In the 3rd intercostal space, 6 cun lateral to the anterior midline of the chest.	Distension and pain in the chest and hypochondrium.
	Zhourong (SP20)	In the 2nd intercostal space, 6 cun lateral to the anterior midline.	①Distension in the chest and hypochondriac regions; ②Cough, asthma.
	Dabao(SP21)	On the mid-axillary line, in the 6th intercostal space.	①Cough, dyspnea; ②Chest and hypochondriac regions; ③Pain of the whole body, weariness of the four limbs.
The Kidney Meridian of Foot-Shaoyin	Yongquan (KI1)	On the sole, in the depression which appears on the anterior part of the sole when the foot is in the plantar flexion , at the junction of the anterior third and posterior two thirds of the line connecting the base of the second and third toes and the heel approximately.	Coma,heatstroke,epilepsy,infantile convulsions, headache, vertigo, dizziness,insomnia, swollen pharynx, aphonia, constipation, dysuria, feverish sensation in the sole.

Name of the meridians	Name of the points	Location	Indications
The Kidney Meridian of Foot-Shaoyin	*Rangu*(KI2)	On the medial border of the foot and in the depression below the tuberosity of the navicular bone, at the junction of the red and white skin.	Irregular menstruation , morbid leucorrhea, prolapsed uterus, seminal emission, impotence, diarrhea, diabetes, difficulty in urination, sore and swollen throat, weakness and flaccidity of the lower limbs, pain instep, tetanus , lockjaw.
	Taixi(KI3)	Posterior to the medial malleolus, in the depression between the tip of the medial malleolus and the calcaneal tendo.	Irregular menstruation, seminal emission, impotence, lumbar pain, cold lower limbs, diabetes, difficulty in urination, constipation, tinnitus, deafness, headache, dizziness, insomnia, forgetfulness, sore and swollen throat, toothache, cough, asthma, pain in the chest, hemoptysis.
	Dazhong(KI4)	On the medial side of the foot, posterior and inferior to the medial malleolus, in the depression anterior to the medial side of the attachment of calcaneal tendon.	Retention of urine, enuresis, constipation, irregular menstruation, hemoptysis, asthma, lumbago, heel pain.
	Shuiquan(KI5)	1 *cun* directly below *Taixi*(KI3), in the depression of the medial side of the tuberosity of the calcaneus.	Irregular menstruation, dysmenorrhea, prolapsed uterus, difficulty in urination.
	Zhaohai(KI6)	In the depression below the tip of the medial malleolus.	Sore and dry throat, red and swollen eyes, insomnia, epilepsy, frequent urination, dysuria, irregular menstruation, dysmenorrhea, morbid leucorrhea, prolapsed uterus.
	Fuliu(KI7)	2 *cun* directly above *Taixi*(KI3), anterior to the achilles tendon.	Edema, night sweat, febrile diseases with anhidrosis or hyperhidrosis, abdominal distension, diarrhea; lumbago, weakness and flaccidity of the lower limbs.
	Jiaoxin(KI8)	On the medial aspect of the lower leg, 2 *cun* above *Taixi*(KI3), 0.5 *cun* anterior to *Fuliu*(KI7), posterior to the medial border of the tibia.	① Irregular menstruation, uterine bleeding, prolapsed uterus; ② Diarrhea, constipation.
	Zhubin(KI9)	On the line connecting *Taixi*(KI 3)and *Yingu*(KI10), 5 *cun* above *Taixi*(KI3), medial and inferior to the gastrocnemius muscle belly.	Psychosis, hernia,vomiting, pain on the medial aspect of the lower leg.
	Yingu(KI10)	With the knee flexed, the point is on the medial side of the popliteal fossa, between the tendons of the semitendinosus and semimembranosu.	Psychosis, impotence, irregular menstruation, uterine bleeding, difficulty in urination, hernia, pain on the medial side of the knee and leg.

Name of the meridians	Name of the points	Location	Indications
The Kidney Meridian of Foot-Shaoyin	Henggu(KI11)	On the lower abdomen, 5 *cun* below the umbilicus, 0.5 *cun* lateral to the anterior midline.	① Pain and distension in the lower abdomen, hernia; ② Seminal emission, impotence, enuresis, difficulty in urination.
	Dahe(KI12)	4 *cun* below the center of the umbilicus, 0.5 *cun* lateral to the anterior midline.	Prolapsed uterus, morbid leucorrhea, irregular menstruation, dysmenorrhea, seminal emission, impotence.
	Qixue(KI13)	On the lower abdomen, 3 *cun* below the umbilicus, 0.5 *cun* lateral to the anterior midline.	① Irregular menstruation, morbid leucorrhea, infertility, impotence, difficulty in urination; ② Diarrhea, dysentery.
	Siman(KI14)	On the lower abdomen, 2 *cun* below the umbilicus, 0.5 *cun* lateral to the anterior midline.	① Irregular menstruation, morbid leucorrhea, seminal emission, enuresis, edema; ② Abdominal pain, constipation.
	Zhongzhu (KI15)	In the center of the abdomen, 1 *cun* below the umbilicus, 0.5 *cun* lateral to the anterior midline.	① Irregular menstruation; ② Abdominal pain, constipation, diarrhea.
	Huangshu (KI16)	In the center of the abdomen. 0.5 *cun* lateral to the anterior midline.	① Abdominal pain and distension, vomiting, diarrhea, constipation; ② Hernia; ③ Lumbar pain.
	Shangqu(KI17)	On the upper abdomen, 2 *cun* above the umbilicus, 0.5 *cun* lateral to the anterior midline.	Abdominal pain, diarrhea and constipation.
	Shiguan(KI18)	On the upper abdomen, 3 *cun* above the umbilicus, 0.5 *cun* lateral to the anterior midline.	① Abdominal pain, vomiting, constipation; ② Infertility.
	Yindu(KI19)	On the upper abdomen, 4 *cun* above the umbilicus, 0.5 *cun* lateral to the anterior midline.	① Abdominal pain and distension, borborygmus, constipation; ② Infertility.
	Futonggu (KI20)	On the upper abdomen, 5 *cun* above the umbilicus, 0.5 *cun* lateral to the anterior midline.	Abdominal pain and distension, and vomiting.
	Youmen(KI21)	On the upper abdomen, 6 *cun* above the umbilicus, 0.5 *cun* lateral to the anterior midline.	Stomachache, vomiting, abdominal distension, and diarrhea.
	Bulang(KI22)	On the chest in the 5th intercostal space, 2 *cun* lateral to the anterior midline.	① Distension and fullness of the chest and hypochondriac regions, cough, asthma; ② Vomiting; ③ Mastiffs.
	Shenfeng (KI23)	On the chest, in the 4th intercostal space, 2 *cun* lateral to the anterior midline.	① Cough, asthma, distension and fullness of the chest and hypochondriac regions; ② Mastitis; ③ Vomiting.

Name of the meridians	Name of the points	Location	Indications
The Kidney Meridian of Foot-Shaoyin	Lingxu(KI24)	On the chest, in the 3rd intercostal space, 2 *cun* lateral to the anterior midline.	①Cough, asthma, distension and fullness of the chest and hypochondriac regions; ② Mastitis; ③ Vomiting.
	Shencang (KI25)	On the chest, in the 2nd intercostal space, 2 *cun* lateral to the anterior midline.	①Chest pain, cough, asthma; ②Vomiting.
	Yuzhong(KI26)	On the chest, in the 1st intercostal space, 2 *cun* lateral to the anterior midline.	Cough, asthma, distending pain in the chest and hypochondriac regions.
	Shufu(KI27)	On the chest, on the lower border of the clavicle, 2 *cun* lateral to the anterior midline.	①Cough, asthma, chest pain; ②Vomiting.
The Liver Meridian of Foot-Jueyin	Dadun(LR1)	On the lateral side of the great toe, 0.1 *cun* lateral from the corner of the toe nail approximately.	Hernia, low abdominal pain, irregular menstruation, metrorrhagia, contraction of scrotum, colpalgia, prolapsed uterus, enuresis, dysuria, hematuria, epilepsy, somnolence.
	Xingjian(LR2)	On the dorsum of the foot, proximal to the web margin between the 1st and 2nd toes, at the junction of red and white skin.	Dizziness, headache, redness, swelling and pain in the eyes, deviation of the mouth and eyes, epilepsy, stroke, distending pain in the chest and hypochondriac region, irregular menstruation, dysmenorrhea, amenorrhea, metrorrhagia, morbid leucorrhea, colpalgia, hernia, enuresis, difficulty in urination, pain in the medial aspect of lower limbs, pain and swelling in the dorsum of foot.
	Taichong(LR3)	On the dorsum of foot, in the depression of the posterior end of the first interosseous metatarsal bones.	Vertigo, headache, redness, swelling and pain in the eyes, tinnitus, angina, deviation of the mouth and eyes, epilepsy, stroke, infantile convulsions, irregular menstruation, amenorrhea, dysmenorrhea, metrorrhagia, morbid leucorrhea, hernia, distending pain in the chest and hypochondriac region, distention in the abdomen, jaundice, vomiting and hiccup, enuresis, dysuria, weakness and flaccidity of the lower limbs, pain and swelling in the dorsum of foot.
	Zhongfeng (LR4)	On the dorsum of foot, 1 *cun* anterior to the medial malleolus, in the depression on the medial side of the tendon of the anterior tibial muscle.	Hernia, seminal emission, difficulty in urination, pain in the abdomen, swelling and pain in the foot and ankle.

Name of the meridians	Name of the points	Location	Indications
The Liver Meridian of Foot-Jueyin	Ligou(LR5)	5 *cun* above the tip of the medial malleolus, on the midline of the medial surface of the tibia.	Irregular menstruation, prolapsed uterus,difficulty in urination, enuresis, pain in the lumbosacral region, hernia.
	Zhongdu(LR6)	7 *cun* above the tip of the medial malleolus,on the midline of the medial surface of the tibia.	Hernia, lower abdominal pain, uterine bleeding, prolonged uterine discharge.
	Xiguan(LR7)	Posterior and inferior to the medial condyle of the tibia, 1 *cun* posterior to *Yinlingquan*(SP9).	Swelling and pain of the knee, atrophy or paralysis of the lower limbs.
	Ququan(LR8)	When the knee is flexed, at the medial end of the popliteal crease posterior to the medial epicondyle of the tibia and in the depression of the anterior border of the insertions of the semimembranous and semitendinous muscles.	Dysmenorrhea, irregular menstruation, prolapsed uterus, morbid leucorrhea, seminal emission, hernia, impotence, difficulty in urination, weakness and flaccidity of the lower limbs, pain and swelling in the knee.
	Yinbao(LR9)	4 *cun* above the medial epicondyle of the femur.	Irregular menstruation, difficulty in urination, enuresis, pain in the lumbosacral region.
	Zuwuli(LR10)	3 *cun* directly below *Qichong* (ST30), inferior to the pubic tubercle.	①Lower abdominal pain and distension, swelling and pain of the testicles, pruritus vulvae, prolapsed uterus, difficulty in urination; ②Scrofula.
	Yinlian(LR11)	2 *cun* directly below *Qichong*(ST30), inferior to the pubic tubercle.	Lower abdominal pain, irregular menstruation, and morbid leucorrhea.
	Jimai(LR12)	Lateral and inferior to *Qichong* (ST30), in the crease of the groin where the femoral artery pulsates, 2.5 *cun* lateral to the anterior midline.	Lower abdominal pain, phallalgia, prolapsed uterus, and hernia.
	Zhangmen (LR13)	Below the free end of the 11th floating rib.	Diarrhea, abdominal distention and pain, vomiting, borborygmus, pain in the hypochondriac region, jaundice, abdominal mass.
	Qimen(LR14)	Directly below the nipple, at the 6th intercostal space, 4 *cun* lateral to the anterior midline.	Distending pain in the chest and hypochondriac region, mastitis, diarrhea, abdominal distention, vomiting, acid regurgitation, hiccup.
The Stomach Meridian of Foot-Yangming	Chengqi(ST1)	On the face, directly below the pupil with the eyes looking straight forward, between the eyeball and the infraorbital ridge.	Trembling eyelids, red and swollen eyes, night blindness, deviation of the mouth and eyes, lacrimation upon exposure to wind.
	Sibai(ST2)	On the face, directly below the pupil with the eyes looking straight forward,in the depression of the infraorbital foramen.	Red, painful itching eyes, blurred vision, trembling eyelids, lacrimation upon exposure to wind, headache and face pain, deviation of the mouth and eyes.

continued

Name of the meridians	Name of the points	Location	Indications
The Stomach Meridian of Foot-Yangming	*Juliao*(ST3)	With the eyes looking straight forward, the point is vertically below the pupil, at the level of the lower border of the ala nasi, on the lateral side of the nasolabial groove.	Deviation of the mouth and eye, twitching at the angle of the mouth, nosebleed, toothache.
	Dicang(ST4)	On the face, 0.4 *cun* beside the mouth angle.	Deviation of the mouth and eyes, trembling mouth angle, toothache, lacrimation.
	Daying(ST5)	Anterior to the mandibular angle,on the anterior border of the masseter muscle, where the pulsation of the facial artery is palpable.	Toothache, deviation of the mouth and eye, swelling of the cheek, facial pain, twitching of the facial muscles.
	Jiache(ST6)	On the cheek, one finger breadth anterior and superior to the mandibular angle, in the depression where the masseter muscle is prominent.	Deviation of the mouth and eyes, swollen cheeks, toothache, locked jaw, spasm of facial muscles.
	Xiaguan(ST7)	On the face, anterior to the ear, in the depression between the zygomatic arch and mandibular notch.	Locked jaw, painful jaw, deviation of mouth, facial pain, toothache, tinnitus, deafness.
	Touwei(ST8)	On the lateral side of the head, 0.5 *cun* above the anterior hairline at the corner of the forehead.	Headache, vertigo,lacrimation upon exposure to wind, trembling eyelids, unclear vision, eyes pain.
	Renying(ST9)	Lateral to the Adam's apple, on the anterior border of m. sternocleidomastoideus, where the common carotid artery pulsates.	①Swollen and sore throat; ②Scrofula, goiter; ③Hypertension; ④Asthma.
	Shuitu(ST10)	On the neck, on the anterior border of m.sternocleidomastoideus, at the midpoint of the line linking the *Renying*(ST9) and *Qishe*(ST11) points.	①Sore throat; ②Cough, gasp; ③Scrofula, goiter.
	Qishe(ST11)	On the neck and on the upper border of the medial end of the clavicle between the sternal and clavicular heads of the sternocleidomastoid muscle.	Swollen and sore throat, scrofula, hiccup, goiter, gasp, pain and rigidity of the neck.
	Quepen(ST12)	In the midpoint of the supraclavicular fossa, 4 *cun* lateral to the anterior midline of the chest.	①Cough, asthma; ②Swollen and sore throat; ③Pain in the supraclavicular fossa; ④Scrofula.
	Qihu(ST13)	At the lower border in the center of the clavicle, 4 *cun* lateral to the anterior midline of the chest.	①Cough, asthma, hiccups; ②Chest pain.
	Kufang(ST14)	In the 1st intercostal space, 4 *cun* lateral to the anterior midline of the chest.	①Cough, asthma; ②Distension and pain in the chest.

Name of the meridians	Name of the points	Location	Indications
The Stomach Meridian of Foot-Yangming	Wuyi(ST15)	In the 2nd intercostal space, 4 *cun* lateral to the anterior midline of the chest.	①Cough, asthma; ②Distension and pain in the chest; ③Mammary abscess.
	Yingchuang (ST16)	In the 3rd intercostal space, 4 *cun* lateral to the anterior midline of the chest.	①Cough, asthma; ②Distension and pain in the chest; ③Mammary abscess.
	Ruzhong (ST17)	In the 4th intercostal space, 4 *cun* lateral to the anterior midline of the chest, at the center of the nipple.	No acupuncture or moxibustion, only as a landmark for locating points on the chest and abdomen.
	Rugen(ST18)	In the 5th intercostal space, vertically below the nipple, 4 *cun* lateral to the anterior midline of the chest.	①Mastitis, insufficient lactation; ②Cough, asthma, hiccups; ③Chest pain.
	Burong(ST19)	On the upper abdomen, 6 *cun* above the center of the umbilicus, 2 *cun* lateral to the anterior midline of the abdomen.	Vomiting, stomachache, abdominal distension, and poor appetite.
	Chengman (ST20)	On the upper abdomen, 5 *cun* above the center of the umbilicus, 2 *cun* lateral to the anterior midline of the abdomen.	Stomachache, vomiting, borborygmus, and poor appetite.
	Liangmen (ST21)	On the upper abdomen, 4 *cun* above the center of the umbilicus, 2 *cun* lateral to the anterior midline of the abdomen.	Stomachache, vomiting, poor appetite, and abdominal distension.
	Guanmen (ST22)	On the upper abdomen, 3 *cun* above the center of the umbilicus, 2 *cun* lateral to the anterior midline of the abdomen.	Abdominal pain and distension, borborygmus, diarrhea, and poor appetite.
	Taiyi(ST23)	On the upper abdomen, 2 *cun* above the center of the umbilicus, 2 *cun* lateral to the anterior midline of the abdomen.	①Abdominal pain and distension; ②Vexation, psychosis.
	Huaroumen (ST24)	On the upper abdomen, 1 *cun* above the center of the umbilicus, 2 *cun* lateral to the anterior midline of the abdomen.	①Abdominal pain, vomiting; ②Psychosis.
	Tianshu(ST25)	2 *cun* lateral to the center of the umbilicus.	Abdominal pain, abdominal distension, borborygmus, dysentery, diarrhea, constipation, intestinal abscess, febrile diseases, edema, irregular menstruation.
	Wailing(ST26)	On the lower abdomen, 1 *cun* below the center of the umbilicus, 2 *cun* lateral to the anterior midline of the abdomen.	①Abdominal pain, hernia; ②Dysmenorrhea.

Name of the meridians	Name of the points	Location	Indications
The Stomach Meridian of Foot-Yangming	Daju(ST27)	On the lower abdomen, 2 *cun* below the center of the umbilicus, 2 *cun* lateral to the anterior midline of the abdomen.	① Lower abdominal distension, difficulty in micturition; ② Spermatorrhea, premature ejaculation; ③ Hernia.
	Shuidao(ST28)	On the lower abdomen, 3 *cun* below the center of the umbilicus, 2 *cun* lateral to the anterior midline of the abdomen.	① Lower abdominal distension, difficulty in micturition; ② Dysmenorrhea; ③ Hernia.
	Guilai(ST29)	4 *cun* below the umbilicus, 2 *cun* lateral to the anterior midline of the abdomen.	Lower abdominal pain, amenia, dysmenorrhea, prolapse of the uterus, leukorrhea, hernia , irregular menstruation.
	Qichong(ST30)	on the lower abdomen, 5 *cun* below the center of the umbilicus, 2 *cun* lateral to the anterior midline of the abdomen.	① Abdominal pain, hernia; ② Irregular menstruation, infertility, impotence, swelling of the vulva.
	Biguan(ST31)	On the line connecting the anterosuperior iliac spine and the superolateral of the patella, on the level of the perineum when the thigh is flexed, in the depression lateral to the sartorius muscle.	Weakness, numbness and pain of the lower limbs, pain of the lower back and leg.
	Futu(ST32)	On the anterior side of the thigh and on the line connecting the anterosuperior iliac spine and the superolateral corner of the patella, 6 *cun* above this corner.	Pain and paralysis of the legs, hernia, abdominal distention.
	Yinshi(ST33)	On the line linking the anterior superior iliac spine and the lower lateral border of the patella, 3 *cun* above the upper lateral border of the kneecap.	Knee pain, atrophy and paralysis of the legs.
	Liangqiu (ST34)	On the anterior side of the thigh and on the line connecting the anterosuperior iliac spine and the superolateral comer of the patella, 2 *cun* above this corner.	Stomachache, knee swelling and pain, mastitis.
	Dubi(ST35)	With the knee flexed, on the knee, in the depression lateral to the patella and its ligament.	Motor impairment of the lower limbs, numbness and pain in the lower limbs, pain in the knees.
	Zusanli(ST36)	On the anterolateral side of the leg, 3 *cun* below Dubi(ST35), one finger breadth(middle finger)from the anterior crest of the tibia.	Stomachache, vomiting, abdominal distension, borborygmus, indigestion, atrophy and pain of the legs, diarrhea, constipation, dysentery, epilepsy, stroke, edema, paralysis of the legs, palpitation, shortness of breath , consumptive disease. This point has the function to strength the body; It is the important point for health care.

Name of the meridians	Name of the points	Location	Indications
The Stomach Meridian of Foot-Yangming	Shangjuxu (ST37)	On the anteriolateral side of the leg, 3 *cun* below *Zusanli*(ST36), one finger breadth(middle finger) from the anterior crest of the tibia.	Abdominal pain and distension, dysentery, constipation, intestine abscess, stroke, paralysis, atrophy and pain of the legs.
	Tiaokou(ST38)	8 *cun* below *Dubi*(ST35).	Atrophy and paralysis of the legs, pain in the abdomen and stomach, pain in the shoulders and arms.
	Xiajuxu(ST39)	3 *cun* below *Shangjuxu*(ST37).	Lower abdominal pain, mastitis, diarrhea, atrophy and paralysis of the legs, diarrhea.
	Fenglong (ST40)	8 *cun* above the tip of the external malleolus, 1 *cun* lateral to *Tiaokou* (ST38).	Sputum, asthma, cough, chest pain, headache, sore throat, constipation, epilepsy, mania, atrophy and paralysis of the legs, vomitting.
	Jiexi(ST41)	In the central depression of the crease between the instep of the foot and leg, between the tendons of the long extensor muscle of the great toe and the long extensor muscle of the toes.	Headache, vertigo, epilepsy, mania, abdominal distention, constipation, atrophy and paralysis of the legs, red eyes.
	Chongyang (ST42)	At the highest point of the dorsum of the foot, between the tendons of m.extensor hallucis longus and digitorum longus, where the dorsal artery of the foot pulsates.	① Stomach pain, abdominal distension; ② Deviation of the mouth, swelling of the face, toothache; ③ Swelling and pain in the dorsum of the foot, weakness and numbness of the foot.
	Xiangu(ST43)	On the dorsum the foot, in the depression distal to the junction of the 2nd and 3rd metatarsal bones.	① Facial and general edema; ② Borborygmus, diarrhea; ③ Swelling and pain of the dorsum of the foot.
	Neiting(ST44)	On the instep of the foot, at the junction of the red and white skin proximal to the margin of the web between the 2nd and 3rd toes.	Toothache, deviation of the mouth and eyes, sore throat, nosebleed, abdominal pain, dysentery, diarrhea, swollen and pain on the instep of the foot, febrile diseases, stomachache, sour regurgitation.
	Lidui(ST45)	On the lateral side of the distal segment of the 2nd toe, 0.1 *cun* from the corner of the toe nail.	Toothache, nosebleed, swollen and sore throat, febrile diseases, profuse dreaming, psychosis.
The Bladder Meridian of Foot-Taiyang	Jingming (BL1)	On the face, in the depression slightly above the inner canthus.	Red and swollen eyes, lacrimation upon exposure to wind, unclear vision, myopia, night blindness, color blindness, blurred vision.
	Cuanzu(BL2)	On the face, in the depression of the medial end of the eyebrow, at the supraorbital notch.	Red and swollen eyes, unclear vision, vertigo, myopia, trembling eyelids, facial paralysis, painful forehead, pain in the supraorbital region.

Name of the meridians	Name of the points	Location	Indications
The Bladder Meridian of Foot-Taiyang	Meichong (BL3)	On the scalp, directly above Cuanzhu(BL2), 0.5 cun within the anterior hairline.	Headache, dizziness, nasal obstruction, epistaxis.
	Quchai(BL4)	On the scalp, 0.5 cun within the anterior hairline, 1.5 cun lateral to the midline. At the junction of the medial one-third and lateral 2/3 of the distance from Shenting(GV24) and Touwei(ST8).	Headache, dizziness, nasal obstruction, epistaxis.
	Wuchu(BL5)	On the scalp, 1.0 cun within the anterior hairline, 1.5 cun lateral to the midline.	Headache, dizziness, epilepsy.
	Chengguang (BL6)	On the scalp, 2.5 cun within the anterior hairline, 1.5 cun lateral to the midline.	Headache, dizziness, nasal obstruction, febrile diseases.
	Tongtian(BL7)	On the scalp, 4.0 cun within the anterior hairline, 1.5 cun lateral to the midline.	Headache, dizziness, nasal obstruction, epistaxis, nasosinusitis, epilepsy.
	Luoque(BL8)	On the scalp, 5.5 cun within the anterior hairline, 1.5 cun lateral to the midline.	Dizziness, blurred vision, tinnitus.
	Yuzhen(BL9)	On the posterior aspect of the head, 2.5 cun superior to the posterior hairline, 1.3 cun lateral to the midline and level with the depression on the superior border of the external occipital protuberance.	Headache and nape of the neck pain, eye pain, nasal obstruction.
	Tianzhu(BL10)	On the nape, 1.3 cun lateral to the midpoint of the posterior hairline, and in the depression of the lateral border of the trapezius muscle.	Headache, dizziness, stiffness of nape, pain in the back and shoulder, nasal obstruction.
	Dazhu(BL11)	On the back, below the spinous process of the 1st thoracic vertebra, 1.5 cun lateral to the posterior midline.	Stiffness of nape, pain in the back and shoulder, cough.
	Fengmen (BL12)	On the back, below the spinous process of the 2nd thoracic vertebra, 1.5 cun lateral to the posterior midline.	Stiffness of nape, pain in the back and shoulder, cough due to wind invasion, fever and headache, nasal obstruction and nose running.
	Feishu(BL13)	On the back, below the spinous process of the 3rd thoracic vertebra, 1.5 cun lateral to the posterior midline.	Cough, asthma, nasal obstruction, chest distress, back pain, tidal fever, night sweating.
	Jueyinshu (BL14)	On the back, level with the lower border of the spinous process of the 4th thoracic vertebra, 1.5 cun lateral to the posterior midline.	①Cardiac pain, palpitations; ②Cough, tightness in the chest; ③Vomiting.

Name of the meridians	Name of the points	Location	Indications
The Bladder Meridian of Foot-Taiyang	Xinshu(BL15)	On the back, below the spinous process of the 5th thoracic vertebra, 1.5 *cun* lateral to the posterior midline.	Cardiac pain, palpitations, restlessness, insomnia, forgetfulness, cough, chest distress, chest pain, epilepsy, night sweating.
	Dushu(BL16)	On the back, level with the lower border of the spinous process of the 6th thoracic vertebra, 1.5 *cun* lateral to the posterior midline.	① Cardiac pain, tightness in the chest; ② Asthma; ③ Stomachache, abdominal distention, hiccups.
	Geshu(BL17)	On the back, below the spinous process of the 7th thoracic vertebra, 1.5 *cun* lateral to the posterior midline.	Stomachache, vomiting, hiccups, tidal fever, night sweating, asthma, hematemesis, urticaria, pruritus.
	Ganshu(BL18)	On the back, below the spinous process of the 9th thoracic vertebra, 1.5 *cun* lateral to the posterior midline.	Jaundice, hypochondriac pain, illness of liver, red eyes, blurred vision, dizziness, epilepsy, mania.
	Danshu(BL19)	On the back, below the spinous process of the 10th thoracic vertebra, 1.5 *cun* lateral to the posterior midline.	Jaundice, hypochondriac pain, bitter taste in the mouth, vomiting, indigestion.
	Pishu(BL20)	On the back, below the spinous process of the 11th thoracic vertebra, 1.5 *cun* lateral to the posterior midline.	Abdominal distention, stomachache, diarrhea, indigestion, vomiting, edema.
	Weishu(BL21)	On the back, below the spinous process of the 12th thoracic vertebra, 1.5 *cun* lateral to the posterior midline.	Abdominal distention, stomachache, indigestion, vomiting.
	Sanjiaoshu (BL22)	On the back, below the spinous process of the 1st lumbar vertebra, 1.5 *cun* lateral to the posterior midline.	Abdominal distention, stomachache, diarrhea, indigestion, vomiting, hypochondriac pain.
	Shenshu (BL23)	On the back, below the spinous process of the 2nd lumbar vertebra, 1.5 *cun* lateral to the posterior midline.	Low back pain, enuresis, difficulty in urination, edema, seminal emission, impotence, irregular menstruation, morbid leucorrhea, dizziness, tinnitus, deafness, asthma, asthenic breathing.
	Qihaishu (BL24)	Level with the lower border of the spinous process of the 3rd lumbar vertebra, 1.5 *cun* lateral to the posterior midline.	① Lumbar pain; ② Dysmenorrhea; ③ Abdominal distention, borborygmus, hemorrhoids.
	Dachangshu (BL25)	On the back, below the spinous process of the 4th lumbar vertebra, 1.5 *cun* lateral to the posterior midline.	Pain of the lumbar and lower limbs, abdominal distention, diarrhea, constipation.

Name of the meridians	Name of the points	Location	Indications
The Bladder Meridian of Foot-Taiyang	Guanyuanshu (BL26)	Level with the lower border of the spinous process of the 5th lumbar vertebra, 1.5 *cun* lateral to the posterior midline.	①Pain of the lumbar region and lower limbs; ②Abdominal distension, diarrhea; ③Frequent urination or difficulty in urination, enuresis.
	Xiaochangshu (BL27)	On the sacrum, level with the 1st posterior sacral foramen, 1.5 *cun* lateral to the median sacral crest.	Seminal emission, enuresis, hematuria, odynuria, morbid leucorrhea, diarrhea, dysentery, hernia, low back pain, sacral pain.
	Pangguangshu (BL28)	On the sacrum, level with the 2nd posterior sacral foramen, 1.5 *cun* lateral to the median sacral crest.	Enuresis, difficulty in urination, low back pain, sacral pain, diarrhea, constipation, seminal emission, morbid leucorrhea.
	Zhonglüshu (BL29)	Level with the 3rd posterior sacral foramen, 1.5 *cun* lateral to the medial sacral crest.	①Diarrhea; ②Stiffness and pain in the lower back; ③Hernia.
	Baihuanshu (BL30)	Level with the 4th posterior sacral foramen, 1.5 *cun* lateral to the medial sacral crest.	①Seminal emission, enuresis, morbid leucorrhea, irregular menstruation, hernia; ②Pain in the lower back.
	Shangliao (BL31)	In the region of the sacrum, between the posterio—superior iliac spine and the posterior midline, in the 1st posterior sacral foramen.	①Irregular menstruation, morbid leucorrhea, prolapsed uterus, seminal emission impotency; ②Difficulty in urination and defecation; ③Pain in the lower back.
	Ciliao(BL32)	On the sacrum, in the 2nd posterior sacral foramen.	Irregular menstruation, dysmenorrhea, morbid leucorrhea, seminal emission, difficulty in urination, hernia, low back pain, sacral pain, weakness or paralysis in the lower limbs.
	Zhongliao (BL33)	In the region of the sacrum, medial and inferior to *Ciliao*(BL32), in the 3rd posterior sacral foramen.	①Irregular menstruation, morbid leucorrhea, difficulty in urination; ②Constipation, diarrhea; ③Lumbosacral pain.
	Xialiao (BL34)	In the region of the sacrum, medial and inferior to *Zhongliao*(BL33), in the 4th posterior sacral foramen.	①Lower abdominal pain, lumbosacral pain; ②Difficulty in urination and defecation, morbid leucorrhea.
	Huiyang (BL35)	In the region of the sacrum, 0.5 *cun* lateral to the tip of the coccyx.	①Diarrhea, dysentery, hematochezia, hemorrhoids; ②Impotency, morbid leucorrhea.
	Chengfu (BL36)	At the midpoint of the transverse gluteal crease.	Pain in the lumbar and legs, weakness or paralysis in the lower limbs, hemorrhoids.
	Yinmen(BL37)	On the line connecting *Chengfu* (BL36) and *Weizhong*(BL40), 6 *cun* below *Chengfu*(BL36).	Pain in the lumbar and legs, weakness or paralysis in the lower limbs.

Name of the meridians	Name of the points	Location	Indications
The Bladder Meridian of Foot-Taiyang	Fuxi(BL38)	On me lateral end of the transverse crease of the popliteal fossa, 1 *cun* above *Weiyang*(BL39) on the medial side of the tendon of the biceps femoris.	① Pain, numbness and spasm in the popliteal fossa and knee; ② Constipation.
	Weiyang (BL39)	On the lateral end of the transverse crease of the popliteal fossa, on the medial border of the tendon of the biceps femoris.	Pain in the lumbar, legs and feet, abdominal distension, difficulty in urination.
	Weizhong (BL40)	On the midpoint of the transverse crease of the popliteal fossa.	Pain in the lumbar, legs and feet, weakness or paralysis in the lower limbs, abdominal pain, acute vomiting or diarrhea, difficulty in urination, enuresis, furuncles, stroke, hemiplegia.
	Fufen(BL41)	On the back, level with the lower border of the spinous process of the 2nd thoracic vertebra, 3 *cun* lateral to the posterior midline.	Stiffness and pain of the neck and back, spasm of the shoulder and back, and numbness of the elbow and arm.
	Pohu(BL42)	On the back, level with the lower border of the spinous process of the 3rd thoracic vertebra,3 *cun* lateral to the posterior midline.	① Cough, asthma, pulmonary phthisis; ② Stiff neck, pain of the shoulder and back.
	Gaohuang (BL43)	On the back, level with the lower border of the spinous process of the 4th thoracic vertebra, 3 *cun* lateral to the posterior midline.	① Cough, asthma, pulmonary phthisis; ② Forgetfulness, seminal emission, night sweats, consumptive disease; ③ Pain of the shoulder and back.
	Shentang (BL44)	On the back, level with the lower border of the spinous process of the 5th thoracic vertebra, 3 *cun* lateral to the posterior midline.	① Cardiac pain, palpitations; ② Cough, asthma, tightness in the chest; ③ Back pain.
	Yixi(BL45)	On the back, level with the lower border of the spinous process of the 6th thoracic vertebra, 3 *cun* lateral to the posterior midline.	① Cough, asthma; ② Malaria, febrile diseases; ③ Pain of the shoulder and back.
	Geguan(BL46)	On the back, level with the lower border of the spinous process of the 7th thoracic vertebra, 3 *cun* lateral to the posterior midline.	① Vomiting, hiccups, belching, dysphagia, tightness in the chest; ② Stiffness and pain of the back.
	Hunmen (BL47)	On the back, level with the lower border of the spinous process of the 9th thoracic vertebra, 3 *cun* lateral to the posterior midline.	① Distending pain in the chest and hypochondrium, vomiting, diarrhea; ② Back pain.
	Yanggang (BL48)	On the back, level with the lower border of the spinous process of the 10th thoracic vertebra, 3 *cun* lateral to the posterior midline.	① Borborygmus, abdominal pain, diarrhea; ② Jaundice, diabetes.

Name of the meridians	Name of the points	Location	Indications
The Bladder Meridian of Foot-Taiyang	Yishe(BL49)	On the back, level with the lower border of the spinous process of the 11th thoracic vertebra, 3 *cun* lateral to the posterior midline.	Abdominal distension, borborygmus, diarrhea, and vomiting.
	Weicang (BL50)	On the back, level with the lower border of the spinous process of the12th thoracic vertebra, 3 *cun* lateral to the posterior midline.	①Epigastric pain, abdominal distension, indigestion; ② Edema.
	Huangmen (BL51)	Level with the lower border of the spinous process of the 1st lumbar vertebra, 3 *cun* lateral to the posterior midline.	①Abdominal pain, abdominal masses; ② Constipation.
	Zhishi(BL52)	Level with the lower border of the spinous process of the 2nd lumbar vertebra, 3 *cun* lateral to the posterior midline.	①Seminal emission, impotence; ②Difficulty in urination, edema; ③Stiffness and pain in the back.
	Baohuang (BL53)	Level with the 2nd posterior sacral foramen, 3 *cun* lateral to the median sacral crest.	①Difficulty in urination, swelling of the vulva;② Abdominal distension, constipation; ③Lumbar vertebral pain.
	Zhibian(BL54)	Level with the 4th posterior sacral foramen, 3 *cun* lateral to the median sacral crest.	①Pain in the lumbar area and legs, atrophy or paralysis in the lower limbs;②Hemorrhoids, constipation, difficulty in urination.
	Heyang(BL55)	On the posterior aspect of the lower leg, 2 *cun* below *Weizhong*(BL40).	Stiffness or Pain in the low back, atrophy or paralysis in the lower limbs, hernia, uterine bleeding.
	Chengjin (BL56)	On the posterior midline of the leg, between *Weizhong*(BL40) and *Kunlun*(BL60), in the center of the belly of the gastrocnemius muscle, 5 *cun* below *Weizhong*(BL40).	Pain in the low back and legs, hemorrhoids.
	Chengshan (BL57)	On the posterior midline of the leg, between *Weizhong*(BL40) and *Kunlun*(BL60), in a pointed depression formed below the gastrocnemius muscle belly.	Pain in the lumbar and legs, hemorrhoids, constipation.
	Feiyang(BL58)	on the posterior aspect of the lower leg, behind the external malleolus, 7 *cun* above *Kunlun*(BL60), 1 *cun* posterior and inferior to *Chengshan* (BL57).	①Pain of the lumbar region and leg;②Headache, dizziness, epistaxis; ③Hemorrhoids.
	Fuyang(BL59)	3 *cun* directly above *Kunlun* (BL60).	Pain in the low back and legs, atrophy or paralysis in the lower limbs, headache.

Name of the meridians	Name of the points	Location	Indications
The Bladder Meridian of Foot-Taiyang	Kunlun(BL60)	Posterior to the lateral malleolus, in the depression between the tip of the external malleolus and Achilles tendon.	Headache, stiffness in the nape, spasm of the back and shoulder, low back pain, heel pain, pediatric epilepsy, delayed labour.
	Pucan(BL61)	On the lateral side of the foot, posterior and inferior to the external malleolus, directly below Kunlun(BL60), lateral to the calcaneus at the junction of the ed and white skin.	①Atrophy or paralysis in the lower limbs, heel pain; ②Epilepsy.
	Shenmai (BL62)	On the lateral side of the foot, in the depression directly below the external malleolus.	Headache, dizziness, stiffness in nape, epilepsy, mania, insomnia, pain in the low back and leg, red and swollen eyes.
	Jinmen(BL63)	On the lateral side of the foot, directly below the anterior border of the external malleolus and below the border of the femur.	①Headache; ②Epilepsy, infantile convulsions; ③Lumbar pain, pain in the lower limbs, pain and swelling in the external malleolus.
	Jinggu(BL64)	On the lateral side of the foot, below the tuberosity of the 5th metatarsal bone, at the junction of the red and white skin.	①Headache, stiff neck, superficial visual obstruction; ②Pain in the lumbar and lower limbs; ③Epilepsy.
	Shugu(BL65)	Posterior to the head of the 5th metatarsal bone, at the junction of the red and white skin.	Headache, stiffness in nape, low back pain, epilepsy.
	Zutonggu (BL66)	On the lateral side of the foot, anterior to the fifth metatarsophalangeal joint, at the junction of the red and white skin.	①Headache, stiff neck, dizziness, epistaxis; ②Psychosis.
	Zhiyin(BL67)	On the lateral side of the distal segment of the little toe, 0.1 cun from the comer of the toenail.	Malposition of fetus, delayed labor, headache, eyes pain, nasal obstruction, nosebleed.
The Gallbladder Meridian of Foot-Shaoyang	Tongziliao (GB1)	Beside the outer canthus, in the depression on the lateral side of the orbital margin.	①Painful and red eyes, cataracts; ②Migraine, deviation of the mouth and eye.
	Tinghui(GB2)	Anterior to the intertragic notch, in the depression posterior to the condyloid process of the mandible when the mouth is open.	Tinnitus, deafness, toothache, deviation of the mouth and eye.
	Shangguan (GB3)	Directly above Xiaguan(ST7), in the depression above the upper border of the zygomatic arch.	Tinnitus, deafness, toothache, facial pain, deviation of the mouth and eye, locked jaw.
	Hanyan(GB4)	In the hair above the temples, at the junction of the upper fourth and lower three fourths of the curved line connecting Touwei(ST8) and Qubin(GB7).	Migraine, vertigo, tinnitus, toothache.

Name of the meridians	Name of the points	Location	Indications
The Gallbladder Meridian of Foot-Shaoyang	Xuanlu(GB5)	In the hair above the temples,at the midpoint of the curved line connecting Touwei(ST8) and Qubin(GB7).	Migraine, red and swollen eyes, toothache.
	Xuanli(GB6)	In the hair above the temples,at the junction of the upper three fourths and lower fourth of the curved line connecting Touwei(ST8)and Qubin(GB7).	Migraine, red and swollen eyes, toothache.
	Qubin(GB7)	At a crossing point of the vertical posterior border of the temples and horizontal line through the ear apex.	Headache, toothache, swelling and pain in the cheek and jaw.
	Shuaigu(GB8)	1.5 cun from the apex of the ear straight into the hairline.	①Migraine, dizziness, tinnitus, deafness; ② Infantile convulsions.
	Tianchong (GB9)	2 cun from the posterior border of the ear straight into the hairline, 0.5 cun posterior to Shuaigu(GB8).	①Migraine, dizziness, tinnitus, deafness;②Goiter;③Fright, epilepsy.
	Fubai(GB10)	At the junction of the central 1/3 and upper 1/3 of the curved line connecting Tianchong(GB9) and Wangu(GB12).	①Migraine, tinnitus, deafness; ②Goiter, scrofula.
	Touqiaoyin (GB11)	Posterior and superior to the mastoid process,at the junction of the middle third and lower third of the curved line connecting Tianchong(GB9) and Wangu(GB12).	Headache, dizziness, stiffness and pain in the neck, tinnitus, deafness.
	Wangu (GB12)	In the depression posterior and inferior to the mastoid process.	①Migraine, tinnitus, deviation of the mouth and eye; ② Stiffness and pain of the neck; ③Epilepsy.
	Benshen (GB13)	0.5 cun above the anterior hairline, 3 cun lateral to Shenting (GV24).	Headache, dizziness, insomnia, epilepsy, infantile convulsions, stroke.
	Yangbai (GB14)	On the forehead, directly above the pupil,1 cun above the eyebrow.	Headache, vertigo, eyes pain, blurred vision, trembling eyelids.
	Toulinqi (GB15)	On the head, directly above the pupil and 0.5 cun above the anterior hairline.	Headache, vertigo, lacrimation, nasal obstruction, infantile convulsion.
	Muchuang (GB16)	1.5 cun within the anterior hairline, 2.25 cun lateral to the midline of the head.	Headache, dizziness, redness, swelling and pain of the eyes, infantile convulsions.
	Zhengying (GB17)	2.5 cun within the anterior hairline, 2.25 cun lateral to the midline of the head.	Headache, dizziness, and epilepsy.
	Chengling (GB18)	4 cun within the anterior hairline, 2.25 cun lateral to the midline of the head.	Headache, dizziness, disease of the eyes, nasosinusifis, and epistaxis.

Name of the meridians	Name of the points	Location	Indications
The Gallbladder Meridian of Foot-Shaoyang	*Naokong* (GB19)	On the lateral side of the superior border of the external occipital protuberance, 2.25 *cun* lateral to the midline of the head.	Febrile diseases, headache, stiffness and pain around neck, dizziness, red and swollen eyes, palpitations, infantile convulsion, epilepsy.
	Fengchi(GB20)	On the nape, below the occipital bone, in the depression between the upper ends of the sternocleidomastoid and trapezius muscles, on the level of *Fengfu* (GV16).	Headache, vertigo, red and swollen eyes, nasal congestion, nasosinusitis, tinnitus, deafness, rigidity and pain in the nape and back, common cold, mania and epilepsy, apoplexy, febrile diseases, common cold, malaria and goiter.
	Jianjing(GB21)	Midpoint linking the line between *Dazhui*(GV14) and the shoulder acromion.	① Pain in the shoulder and upper back, stiffness and pain in the neck; ② Mastitis, insufficient lactation; ③ Delayed labor; ④ Scrofula.
	Yuanye(GB22)	On the axillary line, 3 *cun* below the axilla, in the 4th intercostal space.	① Pain in the hypochondriac region, swelling of the axilla, tightness in the chest; ② Spasm and pain in the upper limbs.
	Zhejin(GB23)	1 *cun* anterior to *Yuanye*(GB22), at the level of the nipple, in the 4th intercostal space.	① Pain in the hypochondriac region; ② Tightness in the chest, asthma; ③ Vomiting, acid regurgitation.
	Riyue(GB24)	Directly below the nipple, 4 *cun* lateral to the anterior midline, in the 7th intercostal space.	① Pain in the hypochondriac region; ② Epigastric pain, vomiting, hiccups; ③ Jaundice.
	Jingmen (GB25)	1.8 *cun* posterior to *Zhangmen* (LR13), on the inferior free end of the 12th rib.	① Difficulty in urination, edema; ② Pain in the hypochondriac region, lumbar pain; ③ Abdominal distension, diarrhea, borborygmus.
	Daimai(GB26)	1.8 *cun* posterior to *Zhangmen* (LR13), at the junction of the vertical line of the free end of the 11th rib and the horizontal line of the umbilicus.	① Irregular menstruation, morbid leucorrhea, amenorrhea, lower abdominal pain; ② Lumbar pain.
	Wushu(GB27)	Anterior to the superior iliac spine, level with 3 *cun* below the umbilicus.	① Irregular menstruation, morbid leucorrhea, prolapsed uterus, lower abdominal pain; ② Pain of the lumbar and hip.
	Weidao(GB28)	Anterior and inferior to the superior iliac spine, 0.5 *cun* anterior and inferior to *Wushu*(GB27).	① Irregular menstruation, morbid leucorrhea, prolapsed uterus, lower abdominal pain; ② Pain of the lumbar and hip.
	Juliao(GB29)	On the midpoint of the line linking the anterosuperior iliac spine and the prominence of the greater trochanter.	① Pain in the lumbar and hip, atrophy or paralysis in the lower limbs; ② Hernia, lower abdominal pain.

Name of the meridians	Name of the points	Location	Indications
The Gallbladder Meridian of Foot-Shaoyang	Huantiao (GB30)	On the lateral side of the thigh, at the junction of the middle third and lateral third of the line connecting the prominence of the great trochanter and the sacral hiatus when the patient is in a lateral recumbent position with the thigh flexed.	Pain in the lumbar area and legs, hemiplegia, and atrophy or paralysis in the lower limbs.
	Fengshi (GB 31)	On the lateral midline of the thigh, 7 *cun* above the popliteal crease, or at the place touching the tip of the middle finger when the patient stands erect with the arms hanging down freely.	Hemiplegia, atrophy or paralysis in the lower limbs, itching of the entire body, beriberi.
	Zhongdu (GB32)	On the lateral side of the thigh, 5 *cun* above the popliteal crease.	Atrophy or paralysis of the lower limbs and hemiplegia.
	Xiyangguan (GB33)	3 *cun* above *Yanglingquan*(GB34), in the depression above the external epicondyle of the femur.	Swelling, pain and spasm in the knee, numbness of the lower leg.
	Yanglingquan (GB34)	On the lateral side of the leg, in the depression anterior and inferior to the head of the fibula.	Pain in the hypochondriac region, bitter taste in mouth, vomiting, hemiparalysis, atrophy or paralysis in the lower limbs, beriberi, jaundice, infantile convulsion.
	Yangjiao (GB35)	7 *cun* above the tip of the external malleolus, on the posterior border of the fibula.	Distention in the chest and hypochondriac region, knee-joint pain, muscular atrophy and weakness of the foot.
	Waiqiu (GB36)	7 *cun* superior to the tip of the external malleolus, on the anterior border of the fibula, level with *Yangjiao*(GB35).	① Distending pain in the chest and hypochondriac region; ② Psychosis; ③ Stiffness and pain in the neck; ④ Atrophy or paralysis in the lower limbs.
	Guangming (GB37)	On the lateral side of the leg, 5 *cun* above the tip of the external malleolus, on the anterior border of the fibula.	Eyes pain, night blindness, atrophy or paralysis in the lower limbs, distention in the chest.
	Yangfu (GB38)	4 *cun* superior to the tip of the external malleolus, slightly anterior to the anterior border of the fibula.	① Migraine, pain in the outer canthus; ② Pain in the chest and hypochondriac region; ③ Scrofula; ④ Atrophy or paralysis of the lower limbs.
	Xuanzhong (GB39)	On the lateral side of the leg, 3 *cun* above the tip of the external malleolus, on the anterior border of the fibula.	Stiffness in the nape, pain and distention in the hypochondriac region, atrophy or paralysis in the lower limbs, sore throat, beriberi, hemiparalysis, hemorrhoid.

Name of the meridians	Name of the points	Location	Indications
The Gallbladder Meridian of Foot-Shaoyang	*Qiuxu*(GB40)	Anterior and inferior to the external malleolus, in the depression lateral to the tendon of the long extensor muscle of the toes.	Stiffness in neck and nape, pain and distention in the hypochondriac region, atrophy or paralysis in the lower limbs.
	Zulinqi(GB41)	On the lateral side of the instep of the foot, in the front of the junction of the 4th and 5th metatarsal bones, in the depression lateral to the tendon of the extensor muscle of the little toe.	Red and swollen eyes, pain in the hypochondriac region, irregular menstruation, enuresis, mastitis, scrofula, malaria, swelling and pain of the dorsum of the foot.
	Diwuhui (GB42)	Between the 4th and 5th metatarsal bones, on the medial side of the tendon of the extensor digitorum longus.	①Headache, redness, swelling and pain of the eye, tinnitus, deafness; ②Mastitis; ③Pain in the hypochondriac region, swelling and pain of the dorsum of the foot.
	Xiaxi (GB43)	Between the 4th and 5th toes, at the junction of the red and white skin, proximal to the margin of the web.	Palpitation, headache, dizziness, tinnitus, deafness, red eye pain, distending pain in the chest and hypochondriac region, swelling and pain in the dorsum of the foot.
	Zuqiaoyin (GB44)	On the lateral side of the distal segment of the 4th toe, 0.1 *cun* from the corner of the toenail.	Headache, red and swollen pain, deafness, sore throat, febrile disease, insomnia, pain in the hypochondriac region, cough, irregular menstruation.
The Conception Vessel	*Huiyin*(CV1)	On the perineum, midway between the anus and the scrotum in men, and the anus and the posterior labial commissure in women.	①Irregular menstruation, difficulty in urination, nocturnal emissions, vaginal pain, pruritus vulva; ②Asphyxiation from drowning, unconsciousness, psychosis.
	Qugu(CV2)	On the anterior midline, 5 *cun* below the umbilicus, in the depression on the midpoint of the upper border of the pubis symphysis.	Difficulty in urination, enuresis, irregular menstruation, dysmenorrhea, morbid leucorrhea, nocturnal emissions, impotence, and eczema of the scrotum.
	Zhongji(CV3)	On the anterior midline, 4 *cun* below the umbilicus.	Dysuria, enuresis, seminal emission, impotence, irregular menstruation, morbid leucorrhea, and infertility.
	Guanyuan (CV4)	On the anterior midline, 3 *cun* below the umbilicus.	Asthenic disease, exhaustion syndrome, seminal emission, impotence, irregular menstruation, dysmenorrheal, morbid leucorrhea, and infertility, dysuria, enuresis; abdominal pain, diarrhea.
	Shimen(CV5)	On the anterior midline, 2 *cun* below the umbilicus.	①Abdominal distension, edema, diarrhea; ②Nocturnal emissions, impotence, uterine bleeding, morbid leucorrhea, difficulty in urination.

Name of the meridians	Name of the points	Location	Indications
The Conception Vessel	Qihai(CV6)	On the anterior midline, 1.5 *cun* below the umbilicus.	Exhaustion syndrome, abdominal pain, diarrhea, constipation; irregular menstruation, dysmenorrheal, morbid leucorrhea, seminal emission, impotence.
	Yinjiao(CV7)	On the anterior midline, 1 *cun* below the umbilicus.	① Abdominal pain; ② Edema; ③ Irregular menstruation, morbid leucorrhea, hernia.
	Shenque(CV8)	In the center of the umbilicus.	Asthenic disease, exhaustion syndrome, abdominal distension, abdominal pain, constipation, diarrhea, edema.
	Shuifen(CV9)	On the anterior midline, 1 *cun* above the umbilicus.	① Edema, difficulty in urination; ② Abdominal pain, abdominal distension, diarrhea, regurgitation.
	Xiawan(CVl0)	On the anterior midline, 2 *cun* above the umbilicus.	Abdominal distension, abdominal pain, diarrhea, vomiting, indigestion; abdominal masses.
	Jianli(CV11)	On the anterior midline, 3 *cun* above the umbilicus.	Stomachache, abdominal distention, loss of appetite, vomiting, edema.
	Zhonwan (CV12)	On the anterior midline, 4 *cun* above the umbilicus, or midway between the umbilicus and the xiphosternal symphysis.	Stomachache, vomiting, acid regurgitation, hiccup, poor appetite, abdominal distention, diarrhea, jaundice, psychosis, epilepsy.
	Shangwan (CV13)	On the anterior midline, 5 *cun* above the umbilicus.	① Abdominal distension, stomach pain, vomiting, acid regurgitation, hiccups, poor appetite; ② Epilepsy.
	Juque(CV14)	On the anterior midline, 6 *cun* above the umbilicus, or 2 *cun* below the xiphosternal symphysis.	① Chest pain, palpitation; ② Psychosis, epilepsy; ③ Stomach pain, vomiting, acid regurgitation.
	Jiuwei(CV15)	On the anterior midline, 7 *cun* above the umbilicus, or 1 *cun* below the xiphostemal symphysis.	① Oppression in the chest, chest pain, palpitation; ② Psychosis, epilepsy; ③ Abdominal distension, hiccups, vomiting.
	Zhongting (CV16)	On the anterior midline, level with the 5th intercostal space, on the center of the xiphostemal symphysis.	① Oppression in the chest, cardiac pain; ② Vomiting, infantile milk regurgitation.
	Danzhong (CV17)	On the anterior midline, level with the 4th intercostal space, or at the midpoint between the nipples.	Oppression in the chest, shortness of breath, chest pain, palpitations, cough, asthma; vomiting, cardiac spasms, lack of lactation.
	Yutang(CV18)	On the anterior midline, level with the 3rd intercostal space.	① Oppression in the chest, chest pain; ② Cough, asthma; ③ Vomiting.
	Zigong(CV19)	On the anterior midline, level with the 2nd intercostal space.	① Cough, asthma; ② Oppression in the chest, chest pain.

Name of the meridians	Name of the points	Location	Indications
The Conception Vessel	Huagai(CV20)	On the anterior midline, level with the 1st intercostal space, at the midpoint of the sternal angle.	① Cough, asthma; ② Distension and pain in the chest and hypochondriac region.
	Xuanji(CV21)	On the anterior midline, on the center of the manubrium of the sternum.	① Cough, asthma, chest pain; ② Swelling and pain in the throat; ③ Dyspeptic disease.
	Tiantu(CV22)	On the anterior midline, at the centre of the suprastemal fossa.	Cough, asthma, chest pain, swollen and painful throat, apoplexy with aphasia, goiter, globus hysterics.
	Lianquan (CV23)	On the neck and on the anterior midline, above the laryngeal protuberance, on the midpoint above the upper border of the hyoid bone.	Swollen sub-lingual region, increased salivation, aphasia with stiff tongue, sudden loss of voice, dysphagia, difficulty swallowing.
	Chengjiang (CV24)	On the face, in the depression at the midpoint of the mentolabial sulcus.	Facial paralysis, swollen gums, salivation, sudden loss of voice, epilepsy.
The Governor Vessel	Changqiang (GV1)	The central point between the tip of the coccyx and the anus below the tip of the coccyx.	Hemorrhoids, prolapse of anus, bloody stool, diarrhea, constipation, psychosis, epilepsy, lumbago, lower back and coccyx pain.
	Yaoshu(GV2)	On the posterior midline, in the sacro-coccygeal hiatus.	① Dysentery, prolapsed anus, constipation, irregular menstruation; ② Lumbago, atrophy or paralysis in the lower extremities; ③ Epilepsy.
	Yaoyangguan (GV3)	On the posterior midline, in the depression below the spinous process of the 4th lumbar vertebra.	Lower back pain, atrophy or paralysis in the lower extremities, irregular menstruation, morbid leucorrhea, nocturnal emissions, impotence.
	Mingmen (GV4)	In the depression below the spinous process of the 2nd lumbar vertebra.	Impotence, seminal emission, irregular menstruation, morbid leucorrhea; lower back pain diarrhea.
	Xuanshu (GV5)	On the posterior midline, in the depression below the spinous process of the 1st lumbar vertebra.	① Stiffness and pain of the lumbar region; ② Abdominal pain, diarrhea.
	Jizhong(GV6)	On the posterior midline, in the depression below the spinous Process of the 11th thoracic vertebra.	① Diarrhea, jaundice, prolapsed anus, hemorrhoids, infantile malnutritional stagnation; ② Epilepsy; ③ Stiffness and pain of the lumbar region.
	Zhongshu (GV7)	On the posterior midline, in the depression below the spinous process of the 10th thoracic vertebra.	① Jaundice; ② Vomiting, distension of the abdomen, stomach pain, poor appetite; ③ Lumbar and back pain.

Name of the meridians	Name of the points	Location	Indications
The Governor Vessel	*Jinsuo*(GV8)	On the posterior midline, in the depression below the spinous process of the 9th thoracic vertebra.	①Epilepsy; ②Vomiting, flaccidity of limbs, spasms; ③Stomach pain.
	Zhiyang(GV9)	In the depression below the spinous process of the 7th thoracic vertebra.	Jaundice, distension and fullness in chest and hypochondriac region, cough, asthma, stiffness of the spine, pain in the back.
	Lingtai(GV10)	On the posterior midline, in the depression below the spinous process of the 6th thoracic vertebra.	①Cough, asthma; ②Furunculosis; ③Stiffness of the spine, pain in the back.
	Shendao(GV11)	On the posterior midline, in the depression below the spinous process of the 5th thoracic vertebra.	①Palpitation, angina, pectoris, amnesia; ②Cough and asthma; ③Stiffness of the spine, pain in the back.
	Shenzhu(GV12)	On the posterior midline, in the depression below the spinous process of the 3rd thoracic vertebra.	①Cough and asthma; ②Fever; ③Headache, stiffness of the spine, pain in the back; ④Back carbuncles; ⑤Epilepsy.
	Taodao(GV13)	On the posterior midline, in the depression below the spinous process of the 1 st thoracic vertebra.	①Cough and asthma; ②Headache; ③Fever, tidal fever, malaria; ④Mania; ⑤Stiffness of the spine, pain in the back.
	Dazhui(GV14)	On the posterior midline，in the depression below the 7th cervical vertebra.	Febrile diseases, malaria, cough, asthma, epilepsy, night sweating, headache, pain in the back and shoulder, stiffness of the lumbar spine, rubella.
	Yamen(GV15)	On the nape, 0.5 *cun* directly above the midpoint of the posterior hairline.	Sudden aphonia, inability to speak due to stiffness of the tongue, mania, epilepsy, headache, stiffness in the neck.
	Fengfu(GV16)	On the nape, 1 *cun* directly above the midpoint of the posterior hairline.	Headache, stiffness in the neck, dizziness, swollen and pain throat, apoplexy with aphasia, mania and epilepsy, hemiplegia.
	Naohu(GV17)	2.5 *cun* directly above the midpoint of the posterior hairline, 1.5 *cun* above *Fengfu*(GV16), in the depression on the upper border of the external occipital protuberance.	①Headache, stiff neck, vertigo; ②Aphonia; ③Epilepsy.
	Qiangjian (GV18)	4 *cun* directly above the midpoint of the posterior hairline, 1.5 *cun* above *Naohu*(GV17) and on the midpoint of the line joining *Fengfu* (GV16) and *Baihui*(GV20).	①Headache, stiff neck, vertigo; ②Psychosis.

Name of the meridians	Name of the points	Location	Indications
The Governor Vessel	Houding (GV19)	5.5 *cun* directly above the midpoint of the posterior hairline, 1.5 *cun* above *Qiangjian*(GV18) or 1.5 *cun* below *Baihui*(GV20).	①Headache, stiff neck, vertigo; ②Psychosis, epilepsy.
	Baihui(GV20)	On the head, 5 *cun* directly above the midpoint of the anterior hairline, at the midpoint of the line connecting the apexes of both ears.	Headache, dizziness, swollen and pain throat, hemiplegia, apoplexy with aphasia, mania and epilepsy, prolapsed anus, prolonged diarrhea, prolapse of uterus, insomnia, forgetfulness.
	Qianding (GV21)	3.5 *cun* directly above the midpoint of the anterior hairline, 1.5 *cun* above *Baihui*(GV20) .	①Headache, vertigo; ②Nasosinusitis;③Psychosis, epilepsy.
	Xinghui (GV22)	2 *cun* directly above the midpoint of the anterior hairline, 1.5 *cun* above *Qianding*(GV21).	①Headache, vertigo; ②Nasosinusitis;③Psychosis, epilepsy.
	Shangxing (GV23)	On the head, 1 *cun* directly above the midpoint of the anterior hairline.	Headache, painful eyes, nasosinusitis, nosebleed, mania and epilepsy, malaria, febrile diseases.
	Shenting (GV24)	0.5 *cun* directly above the midpoint of the anterior hairline .	①Headache, vertigo, nasosinusitis, nosebleed, conjunctival congestion, corneal opacity;②Insomnia; ③Psychosis.
	Suliao(GV25)	At the tip of the nose.	①Nasosinusitis, nosebleed; ②Unconsciousness, apnea, convulsions.
	Shuigou (GV26)	On the face, at the junction of the upper third and middle third of the philtrum.	Coma, syncope, epilepsy, mania and epilepsy, facial paralysis, infantile convulsion, swollen lips and face, stiffness of the lumbar spine.
	Duiduan (GV27)	On the midline, at the junction of the margin of the upper lip and the philtrum.	①Unconsciousness, syncope, psychosis;②Facial distortion, swollen, painful gums, nosebleed.
	Yinjiao(GV28)	In the superior frenulum, at the junction of the upper lip and the gums .	①Facial distortion, swelling and pain of the gums, halitosis, nosebleed nasal obstruction; ②Psychosis.
Extra points	Sishencong (EX-HN1)	This name refers to four points located on the vertex, 0.5 *cun* posterior, anterior and lateral to *Baihui*(GV20).	Vertigo, headache, forgetfulness, insomnia, paralysis, epilepsy, mania.
	Yintang (EX-HN3)	Midway between the medial ends of the two eyebrows.	Headache, vertigo, rhinorrhea, epistaxis, infantile convulsions, insomnia.
	Yuyao (EX-HN4)	Directly above the pupils when the eyes are looking straight forwards, in the center of the eyebrow.	Red and swollen eyes, pain in the supraorbital region, cataract, ptosis of the eyelids, twitching eyelids.

Name of the meridians	Name of the points	Location	Indications
Extra points	Taiyang (EX-HN5)	In the depression about one finger-breadth posterior to the midpoint between the lateral end of the eyebrow and the outer canthus.	Red and swollen eyes, headache, dizziness, wry face and eyes, toothache.
	Erjian (Ex-HN6)	On the top region of the ear, fold the ear forward, the point is at the apex of the ear.	Swollen and painful eyes, hordeolum, swelling and pain in the throat, headache ,vertigo.
	Qiuhou (Ex-HN7)	At the junction of the lateral 1/4 and medial 3/4 of the infraorbital margin.	Eye diseases.
	Shangyingxiang (Ex-HN8)	On the region of the face, at the junction of the cartilage of the ala nasi and nasal concha, near the upper end of the nasolabial groove.	Nasal obstruction, sinusitis, soreness and furuncles in the nasal region.
	Neiyingxiang (Ex-HN9)	Inside of the nostrils, on the mucosal membrane at the junction of the cartilage of the ala nasi and the nasal concha.	Diseases of the nose, inflammation of the throat, swelling and pain in the eyes, febrile disease, sunstroke, vertigo.
	Dangyang (EX-HN11)	Have the patient look straight forward. The point is directly above the center of the pupil, 1 cun within the hairline.	Headache, dizziness and vertigo, congestion in the eye and common cold with nasal obstruction.
	Jinjin (EX-HN12), Yuye(EX-HN13)	In the mouth, on the two veins under the tongue, with Jinjin on the left and Yuye on the right.	Swollen tongue, stiff tongue, ulcers in the mouth, vomiting, aphasia and diabetes.
	Yiming (EX-HN14)	On the neck, 1 cun posterior to Yifeng(SJ17).	Vertigo, headache, diseases of eyes, tinnitus, insomnia.
	Anmian (EX-HN16)	Midway between Yifeng(SJ17) and Fengchi(GB20).	Insomnia, headache, dizziness and vertigo, palpitation, restlessness, hypertension, deafness and hysteria.
	Jingbailao (EX-HN15)	Have the patient sit with the head bent slightly forward, or lie in a prone position. The point is 1 cun lateral and 2 cun above Dazhui(GV14).	Scrofula, cough, asthma, bone-steaming, tidal fever, spontaneous sweating, night sweating, neck rigidity, neck pain, sore throat and general pain after labour due to the invasion of exogenous pathogenic wind and dampness.
	Zigong (EX-CA1)	4 cun below the center of umbilicus, 3 cun lateral to Zhongji (RN3).	Irregular menstruation, uterine bleeding, dysmenorrheal, prolapsed uterus, infertility, hernia.
	Dingchuan (EX-B1)	Below the spinous process of the 7th cervical vertebra, 0.5 cun lateral to the posterior midline.	Asthma, cough, rigidity and pain in the shoulder and back, stiff neck.

Name of the meridians	Name of the points	Location	Indications
Extra points	Jiaji(EX-B2)	0.5 cun lateral to the lower border of each spinous process from the 1st thoracic vertebrae to the 5th lumbar vertebrae. There are 17 points on each side, 34 points on both sides.	There are many indications. The Jiaji points on the upper back are indicated for disorders of the heart, lung and upper limbs, while those on the lower back for disorders of the spleen and stomach, and those on the lumbar region are indicated for disorders of the lumbar region and lower abdomen, and lower limbs.
	Weiwanxiashu (EX-B3)	1.5 cun lateral to the lower border of the spinous process of the 8th thoracic vertebra.	Stomachache, pain in the chest and hypochondriac region, abdominal pain, diabetes, dry throat.
	Pigen(EX-B4)	Blow the spinous process of L1, 3.5 cun lateral to the spinal column.	Abdominal masses, stuffiness and fullness in the chest and abdomen, splenomegaly, hepatomedaly, nephroptosis, hernial pain, lumbar pain and nausea.
	Yaoyan(EX-B7)	In the depression 3.5 cun lateral to the lower border of the spinous process of the 4th lumbar vertebra.	Lumbago, morbid leucorrhea, irregular menstruation, consumptive disease.
	Shiqizhui (EX-B8)	On the posterior midline, in the depression below the spinous process of the 5th lumbar vertebra.	Pain in the lumbosacral region, paralysis of the lower extremities, dysmenorrhea, uterine bleeding, pain and flaccidly of the legs and difficulty in urination.
	Yaoqi(EX-B9)	2 cun directly above the tip of the coccyx,in the depression of the sacral horn.	Constipation, hemorrhoids, epilepsy, headache, insomnia.
	Erbai(EX-UE2)	On the palmar aspect of the forearm, 4 cun proximal to the transverse crease of the wrist, on both sides of the tendon of the m.flexor carpi radialis. Each side has one point, each arm has two points.	Hemorrhoids, Constipation, prolapse of the rectum, pain in the chest and hypochondriac region, pain in the forearm.
	Zhongquan (EX-UE3)	Midway along the line between Yangxi(LI5) and Yangchi(SJ4), in the depression on the radial side of the tendon of m.extensor digitorum communis.	Fullness and distension in the hypochondriac region, cough, asthma, epigastric pain, feverish sensation in the palm, abdominal distention and pain.
	Yaotongdian (Ex-UE7)	On the dorsum of the hand, between the 2nd and 3rd, 4th and 5th metacarpal bones respectively, at the middle points from the line through the metacarpophalangeal joints to the transverse crease of the wrist. There are 2 points on each hand, consisting of 4 points total.	Acute lumbar muscle sprain.

continued

Name of the meridians	Name of the points	Location	Indications
Extra points	*Wailaogong* (EX-UE8)	On the dorsum of the hand, between the 2nd and 3rd metacarpal bones, 0.5 *cun* posterior to the metacarpophalangeal joint.	Stiff neck, stomachache, swelling and redness in the back of the hands, numbness of the fingers.
	Baxie(EX-UE9)	Hand slightly flexed, on the dorsum of hands, in the web between each finger from thumb to little finger, 8 points on the dorsum of both left and right hands.	Swelling and pain on the dorsum of the hand, numbness and spasmodic pain in the interphalangeal joints.
	Sifeng (EX-UEl0)	On the palmar side of the index, middle, ring and little fingers and at the center of the proximal interphalangeal joints.	Infantile malnutrition and pertussis, infantile diarrhea, cough and asthma.
	Shixuan (EX-UE11)	At the tips of the ten fingers, about 0.1 *cun* distal to the nails, 10 acupionts on left and right fingers.	High fever, coma, epilepsy, infantile syncope, sore throat, numbness of the fingers.
	Heding (EX-LE2)	Above the knee, in the depression of the midpoint of the superior patellar border.	Knee pain, weakness of the leg and foot, paralysis of lower extremities,beriberi.
	Baichongwo (EX-LE3)	When the knee is flexed, the point is on the medial aspect of the thigh, 3 *cun* above the medial superior corner of the patella,1 *cun* superior to *Xuehai*(SP10).	Ascariasis, itching of the skin, eczema, rubella, skin ulcers on the lower portion of the body.
	Xiyan(EX-LE5)	When the knee is flexed, in the depression medial and lateral to the patellar ligament. The medial side is also called *Neixiyan* and the lateral side is called *Waixiyan*.	Pain and sourness of the knee joint, and pain and weakness in the lower limbs, beriberi.
	Dannang (EX-LE6)	On the superior lateral aspect of the lower leg, 2 *cun* directly below the depression anterior and inferior to the small head of the fibula *Yanglingquan*(GB34).	Pain in the hypochondriac region, cholelithiasis, acute and chronic cholecystitis, biliary ascariasis, jaundice, pain and weakness of the lower limbs.
	Lanwei (EX-LE7)	On the superior anterior aspect of the lower leg, 5 *cun* below *Dubi*(ST35), one finger-breadth from the anterior crest of the tibia.	Acute or chronic appendicitis, stomachache, poor appetite, weakness and pain of the lower limbs.
	Bafeng (EX-LE10)	On the dorsum of the foot, in the depression between the webbing of the toes, at the junction of the red and white skin, proximal to the web margin.4 points on one side, 8 points totally.	Pain and swelling on the dorsum of the foot, venomous snake bite, beriberi.